Physical Literacy
Throughout the lifecourse

Edited by Margaret Whitehead

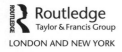
Routledge
Taylor & Francis Group

LONDON AND NEW YORK

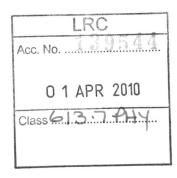
First published 2010
by Routledge
2 Park Square, Milton Park, Abingdon, Oxon OX14 4RN

Simultaneously published in the USA and Canada
by Routledge
270 Madison Avenue, New York, NY 10016

*Routledge is an imprint of the Taylor & Francis Group,
an informa business*

© 2010 selection and editorial material, Margaret Whitehead;
individual chapters, the contributors

Typeset in Sabon
by Keystroke, Tettenhall, Wolverhampton
Printed and bound in Great Britain
by TJ International Ltd, Padstow, Cornwall

British Library Cataloguing in Publication Data
A catalogue record for this book is available
from the British Library

Library of Congress Cataloging-in-Publication Data
A catalog record has been requested for this book

ISBN10: 0–415–48742–0 (hbk)
ISBN10: 0–415–48743–9 (pbk)
ISBN10: 0–203–88190–7 (ebk)

ISBN13: 978–0–415–48742–9 (hbk)
ISBN13: 978–0–415–48743–6 (pbk)
ISBN13: 978–0–203–88190–3 (ebk)

Physical Literacy

What is physical literacy?

What are the benefits of being physically literate?

The term 'physical literacy' describes the motivation, confidence, physical competence, knowledge and understanding that individuals develop in order to maintain physical activity at an appropriate level throughout their life. Physical literacy encompasses far more than physical education in schools or structured sporting activities, offering instead a broader conception of physical activity, unrelated to ability. Through the use of particular pedagogies and the adoption of new modes of thinking, physical literacy promises more realistic models of physical competence and physical activity for a wider population, offering opportunities for everyone to become active and motivated participants.

Physical Literacy is the first book to fully explore the meaning, significance and philosophical rationale behind this important and emerging concept, and the first to apply the concept to physical activity across the lifecourse, from infancy to old age. Including contributions from leading thinkers, educationalists and practitioners, this book is essential reading for all students and professionals working in physical education, sport, exercise and health.

Margaret Whitehead has spent her career in physical education, teaching and lecturing. Her study of existentialism and phenomenology confirmed her commitment to the value of physical activity for all. She has developed the concept of physical literacy over the past ten years and presented on the topic worldwide.

International Studies in Physical Education and Youth Sport

Series Editor: Richard Bailey, University of Birmingham, UK

Routledge's *International Studies in Physical Education and Youth Sport* series aims to stimulate discussion on the theory and practice of school physical education, youth sport, childhood physical activity and well-being. By drawing on international perspectives, both in terms of the background of the contributors and the selection of the subject matter, the series seeks to make a distinctive contribution to our understanding of issues that continue to attract attention from policy-makers, academics and practitioners.

Also available in this series:

x *Contents*

Contributors

Len Almond Ph.D. is Foundation Director of the British Heart Foundation National Centre for Physical Education and Health at Loughborough University. Len was formerly Director of Physical Education at Loughborough University. Following his retirement from this post he took up the chair of the National Coalition for Active Ageing as well as the recently formed National Advisory Group for Early Years. Len is currently working on two projects. He is examining the relationship between low motor ability and inactivity with low academic achievement in children aged 3 to 5 years, and monitoring an intervention to see if increasing energetic play will enhance academic achievement. The second project is to develop a framework for what he calls a pedagogy of engagement and to translate the findings of the first project into practical exemplars for teachers.

Kenneth Fox Ph.D. is Professor of Exercise and Health Science at the University of Bristol. Kenneth has dedicated his career to research and policy development in the field of exercise and health. His books are in exercise psychology and include *The Physical Self: From Motivation to Well-being* (1997, Human Kinetics). He was Senior Scientific Editor of the UK Chief Medical Officer's report on physical activity and health, and serves on the advisory panel for the Cross Governmental Obesity Strategy Unit. He was recently awarded an honorary doctorate by the University of Coimbra in Portugal and is a Fellow of the British Association of Sport and Exercise Sciences, the Physical Education Association, and the American Academy of Kinesiology and Physical Education.

Paul Gately Ph.D. is Carnegie Professor of Exercise and Obesity and Director of Carnegie Weight Management. Paul has a BA in sports science and a M.Med.Sci. Human Nutrition. His primary research interest is childhood obesity treatment strategies. His Ph.D. evaluated and redeveloped an American residential weight loss camp. He runs the successful Carnegie International Camp and Carnegie Clubs throughout Britain. Paul has delivered over 250 keynote presentations and scientific publications and has co-authored seven book chapters. He has a contributed to several policy documents on childhood obesity and is a frequent consultant to government agencies, health organisations and corporations.

Dominic Haydn-Davies M.A. is Senior Lecturer at Roehampton University. Dominic worked as a primary schoolteacher before specialising in primary physical education and working as a School Sport Partnership Development Manager. He now works in initial teacher education, lecturing on a range of courses including the undergraduate specialism in primary physical education. As part of a Best Practice Research Scholarship he developed practical approaches to physical literacy in schools. He currently researches in the areas of teacher education, primary physical education, special educational needs and the early years. Dominic regularly contributes to journals and has been involved in the development and authoring of a number of national resources.

Patricia Maude MBE is a Physical Education Consultant. Patricia is Bye-Fellow at Homerton College, University of Cambridge. Her current research and publication interests include movement development in young children and physical literacy. She is also interested in movement observation and analysis, particularly in relation to teacher education. Recent publications include a chapter on movement development, in *Teaching and Learning in the Early Years* (Whitebread (ed.) 2008, RoutledgeFalmer) and 'How outdoor play develops physical literacy', in the *Early Years Educator Journal*, April 2009. In 2007 she co-authored the DVD and book *A Practical Guide to Teaching Gymnastics* (Coachwise on behalf of afPE), and in 2008 she served on the NICE Programme Development Group on 'Promoting physical activity in children'.

Elizabeth Murdoch OBE is Emeritus Professor at the University of Brighton. Elizabeth retired from the University of Brighton in 1997 and has pursued a role as an education consultant. She was a member of a number of national working parties on physical education, sport and the arts, both in Scotland and England. Elizabeth has published and researched in the area of human movement and learning, with particular reference to both children's development and the art of dance. She has also studied choreutics (movement in space) in relation to understanding how the movement of the body through space can influence both the physical competence of children and adults and choreography in dance theatre.

Karen DePauw Ph.D. is Vice-President and Dean for Graduate Education at Virginia Polytechnic Institute and State University. Karen is also Professor in the Departments of Sociology and Human Nutrition, Foods and Exercise. She has earned an international reputation in the fields of adapted physical education and disability sport, has published extensively, and presented at many international conferences. Karen has served in many leadership roles in professional associations including President of the International Federation of Adapted Physical Activity and the National

Association for Physical Education in Higher Education. Karen was elected as a member of the American Academy for Kinesiology and Physical Education and has received several prestigious awards from professional associations.

Philip Vickerman Ph.D. is Professor of Inclusive Education and Learning at Liverpool John Moores University. Philip is also Head of Research in Physical Education, Sport and Dance and has worked in a range of school and community contexts supporting children and adults with a disability. Philip is a National Teaching Fellow awarded by the Higher Education Academy and has published widely in the field of inclusion, diversity and physical activity.

Margaret Whitehead Ph.D. is a Physical Education Consultant. Margaret retired in 2000 from full-time work at De Montfort University Bedford, where she was Head of Quality for the Faculty of Health and Community Studies. She now works part-time at the University, contributing to PE ITT courses. Margaret taught physical education in school and lectured at Homerton College before moving to Bedford. She has devised, led and taught on a range of initial teacher education courses in physical education. In addition, Margaret studied philosophy of education and completed a Ph.D. on the implications of existentialism and phenomenology to the practice of physical education. In recent years she has developed the concept of physical literacy, running seminars in the UK and reading papers at numerous international conferences.

Foreword

This book is the culmination of years of thought and reflection, grounded in Margaret Whitehead's conviction that dualistic thinking about mind and body is both limiting and damaging. Her conviction threads through the entire book, and the challenge of researching and writing in language which stems from dualist thinking is again and again demonstrated, by the Editor and the various contributors.

As lifelong believers in and advocates for inclusive physical education, we believe that the concept of physical literacy encourages physical educators to place all learners at the heart of the processes of acquiring the levels and sophistication of physical competence and capability, required for effective and efficient engagement in everyday, individual and organised activities; and that teachers' aspirations for pedagogy are enriched and extended by focus on physical literacy as the major outcome of physical education. As the various contributors to this book show, this aspiration is shared, whether learners represent a 'normal' range of abilities and capacities; whether there is a purpose of remediation, compensation or rehabilitation; and irrespective of cultural and social differences.

We witnessed others realising this, during Margaret Whitehead's keynote presentation at the 2001 Congress of the International Association of Physical Education and Sport for Girls and Women, held in Alexandria, Egypt, six weeks after the terrorist attacks on the World Trade Center in New York. Margaret's careful, sensitive offer of the importance of physical literacy for physical educators was enthusiastically received and embraced by her audience, whose members came from all over the globe. It was a wonderful example of a universal concept, whose relevance to physical education pedagogy was immediately recognised by this culturally varied audience, despite language and conceptual differences, and variation of delivery systems. This international interest has been maintained by those practitioners and researchers from all over the world, who visit Margaret's website (www.physical-literacy.org.uk).

Later that year, the importance of Margaret's arguments was reinforced during the National Summit on Physical Education (UK) (see www.ccpr. org.uk), when researchers from a wide range of disciplines, including physical, social and human sciences, each emphasised the value of good quality physical education in developing self-efficacy, self-confidence and self-esteem – all vital elements of physical literacy, as characterised in this book.

Using the outcome of physical literacy as the central aspiration for physical education can liberate physical education from its common, rather limited role as mere servant of sports development, while at the same time improving its effectiveness as an agent of life-long engagement in healthy, enjoyable, meaningful physical activities, physical experience and learning. Such liberation will no doubt be threatening and scary for many physical educators; but it would provide a robust basis for justifying physical education's place in children's (and adults') learning, and in school curricula. It is worth recording that, when discussing a definition for physical education, the use of physical literacy as an outcome is warmly supported by head teachers of primary schools, because it provides such a strong and meaningful analogy with oracy and numeracy as the outcomes of language and mathematics.

Margaret Whitehead, as author, has provided thoughtful, thorough explication of the concept of physical literacy; but she has not been satisfied with this. She has worked intensively with highly experienced practitioners and eminent researchers, to test her ideas and refine her thinking – acts of courage which are all too rare in academic and professional life! As editor, she has sought rigorous examination of the concept and its applicability, from talented contributors who use a wide range of disciplines, experience and interests, asking them to reflect and report on their views of its applicability and relevance. Hence, she seeks to demonstrate the universality of the concept, while ensuring that context and purpose are not ignored – rather, they are used to test physical literacy's relevance to different human beings and different purposes, in different cultural contexts.

Margaret Whitehead and her contributors share with us, their philosophy and application of the concept of physical literacy. They show its relevance, for young persons; and throughout the whole life course, for all people. It becomes evident through the different contributions, that every individual will be on his or her own physical literacy journey, despite differences in ability, culture, gender or social background.

In the context of education, everyone involved is challenged to ensure that each individual is given the opportunity to become a physically literate individual: this includes the development of personal and inter-personal capacities. In this holistic approach, the focus is on learning to move and moving to learn, with confidence and capability. This is an essential and universal aim of teaching and it should be at the heart of every curriculum, in particular in physical education. Several contributors focus on inclusive physical education as an integral part of inclusive education. The education system needs to be designed to embrace and respect diversity. Such an inclusive approach in education enhances the possibility of an inclusive society.

However, as several contributors have discussed, there are problems and issues that need to be addressed. There is as yet, no universal understanding of the importance of physical literacy, and it is therefore essential to develop and implement strategies to promote its understanding and adoption. Margaret Whitehead provides, in her final chapter, an extensive list of recommendations for the way ahead, with identified needs and responsibilities. It is many years since she opened the debate on the concept of physical literacy. She and her contributors have taken us on an exciting journey, challenging readers to rethink their own philosophy and practices, to participate in a new way of thinking about the human being.

This book is an important contribution to thinking and practice (dualist terms, how can we escape them?) in education, therapy, physical education and childhood development. We look forward to seeing its influence on professional development and research in these areas; and most importantly for us, on the experiences of physical education for children across the world.

Margaret Talbot, Ph.D. OBE FRSA
President,
International Council of Sport Science and
Physical Education

Gudrun Doll-Tepper, Prof. Dr. Dr. h.c.
Former President,
International Council of Physical Education
and Sport Science

Acknowledgements

I must start with an acknowledgement of the late Ray Elliott, my Ph.D. supervisor. Without his unfailing interest, challenge and support I would never have started down the road I am now travelling. Would that he was still with us to share in the fruits of his inspiration.

With respect to this text I would like to thank, most sincerely, all those who have worked with me in producing this book. All the co-authors have given most generously of their time. Their willingness to engage in endless debate and their patience in respect of my stream of requests has been remarkable. I would also like to thank all those who have provided case studies for some of the chapters: Claire Hale, Dave Stewart, Claudia Cockburn and Tansin Benn. These contributions are invaluable in bringing physical literacy to life. The support from Margaret Talbot and Gudrun Doll-Tepper in their co-writing of the foreword is much appreciated. I would also like to express my thanks to the Society of Educational Studies which provided funds for a national seminar and a series of workshops, all of which promoted the development of the concept of physical literacy. Sincere thanks are due to all those colleagues who have taken time to engage with me in debate concerning the concept. Their questioning has challenged me to clarify and develop my thinking. Particular thanks are due to Elizabeth Murdoch for her tremendous support throughout the conception and writing of this book. Without her encouragement I doubt if the text would have become a reality. Last but not least I must acknowledge the support of my husband. His enthusiasm for the project and patience have sustained me through the eighteen months of creating the book. I have relied on him totally to ensure that the computer did not swallow any of the scripts. His willingness to drop everything whenever modern technology was against me kept me sane – on more occasions than I would like to admit.

Part I
Philosophical background

1 Introduction

Margaret Whitehead

Motivation to develop the concept of physical literacy

There have been four principal influences that have motivated the development of the concept of physical literacy presented in this book. First and most importantly, the philosophical writings of existentialists and phenomenologists which give significant support for the centrality of embodiment in human existence. Arguing from their particular standpoints, these philosophers see embodiment as fundamental to human life as we know it.[1] Embodiment, in their terms, affords us interaction with our environment and provides the foundation for the development of a wide range of human capabilities. These views were first expressed in the early twentieth century and, interestingly, there is now, some 75 years later, considerable evidence from different fields of science that endorses this view of the fundamental importance of our embodiment in human existence, not least in respect of development in the early years of life. This book provides an opportunity to share some of these more recent findings.

Second was the perception that, despite the views identified above, the importance of movement development in early childhood was being forgotten. The focus that predominated in the early years of education was directed principally towards the development of language, numeracy and social skills. That movement was the foundation for much of child development was not recognised and was not getting the attention it deserved. There is now a great deal of empirical research, for example, as in cognitive science, that supports the fundamental importance of movement development.

Third is the widespread unease about the growing drift away from physical activity as part of our lifestyle, particularly in developed countries. A decrease in physical activity can, unfortunately, exacerbate the problems of obesity and poor physical and mental health. Philosophical underpinning supports the view that physical activity can enrich life throughout the lifecourse. There had previously been a view that physical activity was most appropriate for younger people. Research has now shown that this is not the case, and that continued involvement in physical activity can have significantly beneficial effects for adults, including the older adult population.

Fourth, there was a growing unease with the general direction that physical education in school in many developed countries, including the UK, was taking – this being very much towards high-level performance and elitism. One result of this focus was the tendency to neglect those pupils who did not have outstanding ability. The notion of participation as valuable in itself was becoming less evident in much work in school, with the consequence that the non-gifted were becoming disillusioned with the subject and often looked for opportunities not to take part. The views of philosophers from the schools of existentialism and phenomenology were convincing in advocating the value of physical activity for all – not just the most talented in this area; hence the need to adopt a new perspective on physical education and to encourage the profession to review its priorities.

Why 'physical literacy': the need to develop the concept

Over the past ten years during which the concept of physical literacy presented in this book has been developed, discussed and shared with many interested parties, the need for developing an additional concept in the field of physical activity that identifies its core purpose and value has been questioned.[2] The underlying reason for this need grew from coming to understand the work of certain philosophers who adopted a particular perspective on our embodied dimension. Looking at human life from a monist perspective they put forward a strong case for the centrality of our embodied nature in very many aspects of human existence. Embodiment influenced life not only as an instrument that can be used for overtly functional purposes but also as an underlying capability that contributes to, for example, cognitive and emotional development. Our embodiment therefore could not be, on their terms, dismissed as a somewhat inferior adjunct to human life. Taking this view of an essentially embodied existence, it was evident that there was no adequate word to describe the very broad potential that the embodied dimension has to contribute to enriching the lives of every individual throughout the whole of the lifecourse; hence the identification of the concept of physical literacy as a significant human capability.

Descriptions of effective deployment of our embodied dimension currently in use include such terms as physically able, strong, able-bodied, skilful, fit, healthy, good at sport, well coordinated and physically educated. All these terms focus on the 'body' as an object and on the deployment of the 'body' as object or instrument in functional situations such as manual work and in the sports context. None of these descriptions looks beyond our 'body' as a machine and most point to a specific group of talented people with the inference that others cannot match up to the description. Moreover, these descriptions seem to implicate that the responsibility for developing our embodied potential rests purely with practitioners in the fields of physical education and sports coaching. Attention to this aspect of our personhood was, therefore, not of interest to, or the responsibility of, those outside these professions.

As a result of the terminology used, descriptions of embodied potential tended to be focused mainly on school-age children, young people and those with particular talent. That every individual was endowed with a valuable embodied capability was ignored. Indeed there was a sort of finality about reaching any of the above goals, such as 'good at sport' or 'physically educated'. It appeared that these were end states that, if not achieved by a certain age or stage, were beyond an individual's reach. In short, most terms used with reference to our embodied capability were dualistic, focused on the young, had a finality about them and were, to some extent, elitist. In contrast to these descriptions physical literacy is described as a capability all can develop. It is a universal concept applicable to every individual whatever their age or physical endowment. The short definition of physical literacy in this text explains:

> *As appropriate to each individual's endowment, physical literacy can be described as the motivation, confidence, physical competence, knowledge and understanding to maintain physical activity throughout the lifecourse.*

Building from the definition above, with the underlying support of some schools of philosophy and scholars in other fields, the notion of physical literacy can:

- identify the intrinsic value of physical activity;
- overcome the need to justify physical activity as a means to other ends;
- provide a clear goal to be worked towards in all forms of physical activity;
- underwrite the importance and value of physical activity in the school curriculum;
- refute the notion that physical activity is an optional extra of only recreational value;
- justify the importance of physical activity for all, not just the most able in this field;
- spell out a case for lifelong participation in physical activity;
- identify the range of significant others who have a part to play in promoting physical activity.

Is 'physical literacy' an appropriate term?

The term 'physical literacy' was decided on as being the most appropriate for a number of reasons. First, there was nothing exclusive about the term. Every individual has, by nature, a physical or embodied dimension. Second, the notion of 'literacy' was also helpful as it is a concept commonly used to describe a human characteristic that it is accepted is within the grasp of most people. Third, the term retained the connection with our physicality but moved the focus away from a narrow performance base to include a more interactive flavour. This is very much in line with the philosophical thinking which argued strongly that we are, as human beings, in constant dialogue with our surroundings.

It is not surprising, however, that in the melting-pot of lively debate the concept of physical literacy has been questioned. Both the words 'physical' and 'literacy' have been contested. 'Physical' was seen to be perpetuating the idea of the 'body' as an object, and 'literacy' was seen as being too closely related to the ability to read and perhaps not a term that it was appropriate to use in relation to our embodied capability.

Alternatives to 'physical' are, first, 'movement'. While it is the case that movement education has often been suggested as an alternative to physical education, the term 'movement' applies to a myriad of non-human phenomena and thus it has not, generally, been seen as appropriate – although it has been used on occasion to describe the physical activity undertaken in education in the early years. Other alternatives to 'physical' are the philosophical terms 'embodied' and 'motile'. Resultant terms would be either 'embodied literacy' or 'motile literacy'. While these might be acceptable terms in the context of philosophy, they were seen as inappropriate for general use, being unfamiliar and somewhat esoteric in nature. Thus, while accepting that the continued use of the term 'physical' has unfortunate associations with dualism, rather than helping to signal the monist view that as humans we are a whole, it was seen to be the most acceptable term to describe our embodied capability.

Suggested alternatives to 'literacy' were 'competence', 'ability' and 'skill'. However, 'physical competence', 'physical ability' and 'physical skill' would seem to leave the concept very much tied to pure physicality and to perpetuate dualistic attitudes. While physical competence forms a key element of physical literacy, the above terms would seem to focus very much on the instrumental use of our embodiment and do not encompass the range of attributes that make up the concept.

The concept of 'literacy' is seen as most appropriate as it:

- moves away from a dualistic approach;
- encompasses doing, interpreting, responding and understanding, thus aligning with monism;
- has holistic associations that readily absorb aspects of human cognition and emotion;
- signals an interplay with our surroundings, which is a critical aspect of the philosophical thinking on which the concept of physical literacy is based;
- has non-exclusive connotations, indicating that everyone can achieve this attribute at their own level.

The concept of literacy is more readily appreciated as relevant to the individual as an essentially holistic embodied being. Physical literacy shares some aspects of notions discussed by other writers such as Best (1978: 58) and Arnold (1979: 17) who refer, respectively, to 'kinaesthetic intelligence' and 'intelligent action', and is, I believe, a much richer and more far-reaching concept than physical competence or physical skill.

It is interesting to note that the term 'physical literacy' is already being used by a range of groups. One of the reasons behind the production of this book is to set out the full definition of the concept in order to clarify its nature. In some cases the term is being used to pick out a particular aspect of the concept. For example, there are instances where physical literacy is being used as a term to describe fundamental movement skills or physical fitness. Another use of the concept focuses on the ability to 'read a game', and yet another use highlights the ability to talk about, describe and write about movement. Each of these interpretations of physical literacy is of value in that each picks out an element of the concept; however, none encompasses the totality of the meaning of being physically literate. As will be seen in Chapter 2, these aspects of physical literacy are included, respectively, in sections B, C and F of the full definition. In another adoption of the concept it has been used to describe a goal for children from 0 to 12 years of age to achieve, rather than an attribute that is pertinent to the full lifecourse. While experiences at this early age are particularly important, the nature of physical literacy means that this capability should be nurtured beyond the earlier years, through maturity and old age.

Questions have also been asked as to how physical illiteracy could be described. From one perspective every human is a physical being and exists only because each is, by nature, embodied. In this context everyone, by definition, has and employs physical competence. However, physical literacy only develops when this dimension is deployed beyond what might be called subsistence level. Physically illiterate individuals will avoid any involvement in physical activity in all situations wherever alternatives are possible. This could include not walking short distances, avoiding tasks such as house cleaning and gardening, preferring quick methods of preparing a meal and always using the remote control to turn on an electrical appliance. Individuals will not be motivated to take part in structured physical activity and will therefore not achieve any refinement or development of their physical competence. They will have no confidence in their ability in the field of physical activity, anticipating no rewarding feedback from such involvement. Individuals will have a very low level of self-esteem with respect to this aspect of their potential and will avoid all inessential physical activity in order to guard against failure and humiliation.

The structure of the book

The book is designed to introduce readers to the concept of physical literacy and to make a case for the adoption of this notion as a goal for all to achieve and maintain throughout life. The philosophical foundations for the concept are explained, as well as recent findings from within the scientific field. This is followed by a consideration of physical literacy in the context of wider issues such as the development of self-esteem, the problem of obesity and the challenge of individual differences. Implications for physical activity work in school and beyond are debated, as are the needs of particular populations. The authors and co-authors of these chapters are specialists within their own fields who have found the concept of physical literacy relevant to their work.

The book is divided into three parts. Part I considers the philosophical background to the approach taken throughout the book and thus the rationale behind the concept. Chapter 2 presents and discusses in detail the concept of physical literacy. Chapter 3 looks in more depth at the philosophy that underpins the concept, with particular reference to the views of existentialists and phenomenologists. The role of our embodied dimension in perception and action is explained. The fundamental view here is that human embodiment is a defining aspect of being and sets the parameters to many aspects of existence. Chapter 4 considers the significance of physical literacy for every individual, whatever their embodied endowment, age or the parent culture within which they live. Chapter 5 proposes aspects of physical competence that can be developed as individuals proceed on their physical literacy journey and then looks at the philosophical arguments that support the importance of effective relationships with the world. Chapter 6 presents the philosophical arguments surrounding the view that physical literacy plays a central role in the development both of a sense of self and of effective interpersonal relationships. It also considers the place of propositional knowledge in the concept.

Part II considers ways that physical literacy connects with issues in a range of specific contexts. Chapter 7 reflects on physical literacy in relation to the physical self. Central here is the attitude individuals have to their embodiment. Chapter 8 looks at physical literacy and obesity. This discussion is presented in the context of current lifestyle trends in Western society. The two following chapters look at, respectively, the importance of physical literacy to the young child and the older adult population. Chapter 9 sets out the relationship between physical literacy, the maturation process and movement development. It also discusses the importance of play as providing opportunities for physical literacy to be fostered in the early years. Chapter 10 focuses on the older individual. This includes discussion of the importance of physical literacy to the realisation of lifelong health and well-being. The problems of inactivity are discussed as well as the values of continuing with appropriate forms of physical activity throughout the lifecourse. Chapters 11 and 12 focus on particular populations – that is, groups of individuals who may encounter difficulties in developing and maintaining physical literacy. Work with people with a disability is discussed in Chapter 11. A range of cases studies are provided and there is debate about how these individuals can be supported within and outside school. Chapter 12 addresses physical literacy and issues of diversity: gender, sexual orientation, religion and culture are considered briefly.

Part III has a more practical focus and contains four chapters. Chapter 13 draws together the principal themes of the book and highlights the role of all significant others in promoting physical literacy. It then looks specifically at the relationship of physical literacy to the structured physical activity that takes place within compulsory education. In the UK these lessons are entitled physical education; however, the debate is relevant in educational contexts worldwide – whatever the title of the work in school. At root this argues that physical literacy is the fundamental goal of school-based physical activity. Physical literacy is seen to challenge those working in this area to return to the roots of physical education in promoting confident participation by all, rather than seeing the subject as principally nurturing the performances of the most able. It argues that this structured physical activity in compulsory schooling is the only, and indeed the unique, opportunity available to ensure that *all* young people develop physical literacy.

Chapters 14 and 15 build from this chapter and consider, first, learning and teaching approaches and then content in school-based physical activity programmes. Chapter 14 looks in detail at the significance of the methods of teaching adopted by teachers for the development of physical literacy by *all* young people. Chapter 15 sets out an overview rationale for the nature of the content of school-based physical activity programmes in the interests of *all* pupils attaining and maintaining physical literacy. This covers curricular and extra-curricular work. Readers are encouraged to critically evaluate the physical activity content currently being delivered in school.

The concluding chapter draws together the philosophical debate in Part I, the insights of specialists from a variety of different fields presented in Part II and the practical implications from Part III. Strategies that need to be adopted to promote the acceptance and establishment of physical literacy as a lifelong goal are suggested, and challenges are set out to different constituencies in respect of their role in this enterprise.

Recommended reading is suggested for each chapter and possible topics for discussion points may be found at the back of the book. Further papers that relate to some chapters in the book may be found on the website www.physical-literacy.org.uk. Papers will be added to the website as the concept continues to develop. In addition some of the tables in the book are available on the website.

2 The concept of physical literacy

Margaret Whitehead

Introduction

This chapter starts with a brief discussion of how the concept of physical literacy relies on a new perspective being taken on our embodied dimension. The detail of the concept is then set out and the relationship between its different attributes explained. The identification of physical literacy as a capability and of the premises that underpin this capability conclude the chapter. Overall, the chapter sets the scene for a more detailed philosophical discussion in Chapter 3.

The need for a new perspective to be taken on our embodied dimension

The use of the concept of physical literacy requires there to be a realignment and a rethinking of attitudes to our embodied dimension and thus the development of a new perspective on this aspect of our human nature. In some instances this will mean the creation of new terminology and possibly the introduction of a new discourse with respect to this human capability.

In Western cultures our embodied dimension is generally considered in its concrete, observable form as a 'thing' or physical object. Reference to this human dimension usually refers to 'its' physical condition or 'its' performance. There is a 'taken-for-granted' attitude that this is the beginning and end of our embodiment. Everyday language, arising from dualistic thinking, persistently refers to the 'body' as an object and so perpetuates the above characterisation of this human dimension. The importance of physical activity is seen predominantly as realised in manual work, participation in culturally designed specific physical activity settings, usually at a high level, and as contributing to physical fitness. It is not surprising, then, that the value given to our embodied dimension in education and life management generally focuses on 'its' role as an instrument in work, elite sports participation and health maintenance. Other deployment of our embodied dimension is often viewed as of no real significance. This is particularly the case in relation to participation in structured physical activities, such as competitive sports at non-elite levels, involvement being viewed as inessential, of little worth and purely for recreation. Therein currently rest both the generally accepted conception of our embodied dimension as an object or instrument and the commonly held view of 'its' value and significance.

However, this is far from the complete picture. To these generally uncontested attitudes to our 'body', or our embodiment, there needs to be added an appreciation of a more fundamental aspect of our nature as embodied beings. This is the ongoing involvement of the embodied dimension in very many aspects of the expression of human life as we know it. As will be seen from the chapters that follow, many philosophers, psychologists and sociologists now refer to this aspect of our embodiment as the body-as-lived or the lived embodiment. The lived embodiment predominantly functions on a pre-reflective or pre-conscious level, and on that account has long been overlooked. However, writers working since the mid-twentieth century have revealed the all-pervading significance of our lived embodiment and this insight has been the principal rationale behind the development of the concept of physical literacy. Physical literacy is thus the human potential that springs from our nature as embodied beings. It is a potential that encompasses the embodiment-as-lived as well as the embodiment-as-object.

The concept of physical literacy brings to the fore previously neglected contributions that our embodied dimension makes to human existence, and throws new light on the nature and importance of our ability to move or motility. The concept lays the ground for a clearly articulated argument for the importance of attention to be paid to this dimension of our nature, in the early years, in adulthood and through to older age. The concept of physical literacy provides a structure within which the significance of the lived embodiment can be identified, understood and appreciated, alongside the embodiment as an instrument. Physical literacy confirms our embodiment as a fundamental aspect of our nature – and in addition reinforces the holistic nature of the human condition.

The creation of new terminology and possibly a new discourse is challenging in that it will need to marry commonly used dualist language with monist principles, with the intention of describing a human capability that clearly demonstrates our holistic nature. That individuals can and do view their embodiment as an object or instrument must not hide the ways that, at a pre-reflective and pre-conscious level, the lived embodiment is central in making us the human beings that we are.

Definition of physical literacy

The concise definition of physical literacy is as follows:

> As appropriate to each individual's endowment, physical literacy can
> be described as the motivation, confidence, physical competence,

knowledge and understanding to maintain physical activity throughout the lifecourse.

In more detail the concept is seen to encompass the following attributes. These attributes have been built up as research into the area has proceeded. The sections below – A to F – describe attributes exhibited by a physically literate individual. Aa is a rider to A and argues that the capability to be physically literate is relevant to all individuals throughout their lifecourse and whatever the culture in which they live.

A. Physical literacy can be described as a disposition characterised by the motivation to capitalise on innate movement potential to make a significant contribution to the quality of life.

Motivation to take part in physical activity is a fundamental attribute in being physically literate.

Physically literate individuals have a positive attitude towards their own embodied dimension, confidence in their physical abilities, carry out everyday tasks with ease and take part in physical activities, secure in the knowledge that this will be a positive and rewarding experience. Being physically literate prolongs an active life and involvement in physical activity adds to the overall quality of life. Physically literate individuals maintain this positive attitude towards physical activity throughout their lifecourse and are involved in a range of different and appropriate forms of physical activity as maturity and old age are reached. Elderly people who are physically literate characteristically retain their independence longer than those who are less active. Physical literacy is a lifelong asset, enriching life at all ages.

Aa. All human beings exhibit this potential. However, its specific expression will depend on individuals' endowment in respect of all capabilities, significantly their movement potential, and will be particular to the culture in which they live.

Physical literacy is a universal concept, applicable to everyone, whenever and wherever they may live. Individuals' age, overall endowment and the extent of their embodied abilities, as well as the culture within which they live, will, of course, influence the specific nature of their physical literacy. There will be different challenges and opportunities in every culture both in respect of the demands of everyday living and in relation to culturally recognised forms of structured physical activity. As human beings we are all in the world in an 'embodied form'. The particular world in which individuals live will foster particular deployment of their embodied capability. However, all individuals can develop and enhance their physical literacy and benefit from the growth of this capability.

B. Individuals who are physically literate will move with poise, economy and confidence in a wide variety of physically challenging situations.

Physically literate individuals will manage their embodied dimension with assurance. This will include overall body management, which might be described as moving with grace or poise. Key capacities here are coordination and control, which will be demonstrated both in whole body action such as travelling, balancing and jumping as well as in finer movements such as handwriting and playing a musical instrument. Physically literate individuals will have developed their capacities in a range of environments, laying the ground for the fluent interaction with numerous and varied settings as described in C below. These embodied abilities enable individuals both to respond to the demands of everyday living and to enjoy opportunities to take part in a range of physical activities.

C. Physically literate individuals will be perceptive in 'reading' all aspects of the physical environment, anticipating movement needs or possibilities and responding appropriately to these with intelligence and imagination.

A physically literate individual can interact fluently with the environment in the context of everyday living and of physical activities. Building on the physical competence alluded to above, which will have been developed in varied settings, the individual will be able to respond appropriately to demands that are encountered, whether they are commonplace or novel. Interacting effectively with our surroundings is satisfying and rewarding.

D. These individuals will have a well-established sense of self as embodied in the world. This, together with an articulate interaction with the environment, will engender positive self-esteem and self-confidence.

Through rewarding experiences of physical activity, the physically literate individual can develop a positive sense of self as well as self-confidence. This positive sense of self is derived from the rewarding experience of effective embodied interaction with the environment. In a sense individuals become fully aware of and 'comfortable with' their embodied nature and embrace this dimension of self as a significant part of their personhood. Furthermore, because of the ways in which physical ability contributes to a wide range of other human attributes, such as language, cognition and rationality, the individual can grow in global self-confidence and self-esteem.

E. Sensitivity to and awareness of embodied capability will lead to fluent self-expression through non-verbal communication and to perceptive and empathetic interaction with others.

Physically literate individuals have confidence in their embodied dimension, receiving positive feedback from this aspect of self. This alert and affirming awareness and experience of self is used to support expression via non-verbal communication. As an outcome of the ability to use their embodied dimension confidently in expressing themselves, these individuals can effect an empathetic relationship with others. Physically literate individuals can readily sense what another is feeling and so can respond with support and understanding. This interpersonal interaction is evident in all areas of life.

F. In addition, physically literate individuals will have the ability to identify and articulate the essential qualities that influence the effectiveness of their own movement performance, and will have an understanding of the principles of embodied health with respect to basic aspects such as exercise, sleep and nutrition.

Physically literate individuals are sensitively aware of their embodied dimension and can reflect astutely on their movement experiences. This embodied awareness enables them to describe and evaluate their own movement as well as engage in a discussion about how their movement can be enhanced. In addition, individuals can assess the effects of exercise on their lifestyle. They can use the experiences of a range of physical activities, and knowledge of related aspects such as diet, to come to understand the impact of activity on all-round health and well-being. Physical literacy, therefore incorporates a rational, informed grasp of our human situation.

The relationships between the attributes of physical literacy

These relationships are best described in two stages. Motivation, confidence and physical competence, and effective interaction with the environment are the three attributes that form the kernel of the concept and are mutually reinforcing.

Figure 2.1 shows the interrelationships between these three attributes of physical literacy. Their reciprocal relationships may be described as follows:

- Motivation (A) can encourage participation and this involvement can enhance confidence and physical competence (B). The development of this confidence and competence can in turn maintain or increase motivation.
- Development of confidence and physical competence (B) can facilitate fluent interaction with a wide range of environments (C). This effective relationship with the environment, with the new challenges this presents, can in turn enhance confidence and physical competence.

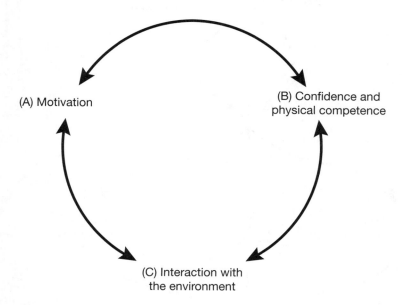

Figure 2.1 The relationship between the key attributes of physical literacy.

- The success of developing effective relationships with a range of environments (C) can add to motivation (A). This enhanced motivation can in turn encourage exploration and promote effective interaction with the environment.

Figure 2.2 shows the relationships between all the attributes. As can be seen, the other three attributes (D, E and F) characteristically develop as motivation, confidence, physical competence and fluent interaction grow. For example, as individuals have rewarding experiences in physical activity they can experience a positive sense of self and enhanced global self-confidence (D). In addition, awareness of the embodied dimension alongside a sound self-esteem will promote fluent self-expression and perceptive and empathetic interaction with others (E). Knowledge and understanding (F) will be enriched by all aspects of participation.

Figure 2.2 also shows how these three attributes (D, E and F) can help to further the core attributes of motivation, confidence, physical competence and fluent interaction with the environment. For example, an assured sense of self will feed into motivation and the willingness to accept challenges, while fluent interaction with others will add to confidence and the ability to work alongside others in physical activity settings. Similarly, knowledge and understanding will support the appreciation of developing physical competence and the perception of different environments.

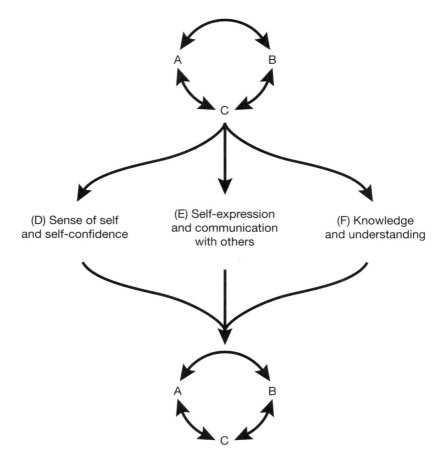

Figure 2.2 The relationship between all the attributes of physical literacy.

The physically literate individual

It may be useful to move from this rather formal description of the characteristics of a physically literate individual, as set out above, to the description of the real-life person. Physical literacy will be evident both in very many aspects of everyday living and in interaction with others, as well as in specific physical activity settings.

Physically literate individuals will present themselves with assurance and self-confidence. They will demonstrate a sense of poise in their movement, coupled with an alert yet thoughtful approach. Within the potential of their physical endowment, individuals will have sound coordination and control, and a sensitive awareness of all aspects of their motility. Individuals will be at ease with themselves as embodied and will have accepted their physical potential. Positive feedback from successful embodied activity will reinforce their confidence and enjoyment in the deployment of their movement abilities. The individual will be able to respond intelligently to the changing context of movement, whether this is related to the movement of others or to objects and features in the environment. Success in the movement area will tend to enhance self-confidence and self-esteem. This positive sense of self will be reinforced by the rewarding experience of effective embodied interaction with the environment. Physically literate individuals will relate to others with ease, demonstrating sensitivity to the non-verbal communication they themselves are exhibiting, as well as that displayed by others. In this way the individual will have an empathetic relationship with others.

Physically literate individuals will enjoy physical activity, being keen to participate, and confident in the knowledge that they will have some success. They will be happy to practise, to try out new activities, and will welcome advice and guidance. They will have an acute awareness of their movement experiences and be able to describe and articulate the various aspects of their movement and discuss ways to improve. The individual will understand the importance of physical activity to lifelong health and well-being, and will readily talk about these issues. The individual will advocate and promote involvement in physical activity in discussion with others and will be able to look ahead through the lifecourse in the expectation that participation in various forms of physical activity will continue to be a part of life. The individual will appreciate the intrinsic value of physical activity, as well as its contribution to health and well-being. Participation will be valued for the pleasure and fulfilment it brings as well as for the challenge and personal development that it offers.

Physical literacy as a capability

Throughout this text physical literacy is referred to as a capability, this being a potential all human beings possess. Physical literacy as a capability describes the expression of our embodied dimension as one aspect of our innate human nature. As human beings, we comprise a range of dimensions through which individuals can interact with the world. On this definition the deployment of each dimension can be described as a particular capability. The identification of different aspects of our human nature in no way militates against the monist principles that are advocated in this text. As is explained below, each person comprises an irrevocably interconnected system of dimensions.

There have recently been two approaches that support this view of multiple dimensions of human beings. One is suggested by Martha Nussbaum (2000) and the other by Howard Gardner (1993). Nussbaum refers to the expression of these aspects of human nature as 'capabilities' while Gardner describes them as 'intelligences'. Nussbaum (2000: Frontispiece) identified ten human capabilities described as 'what people are actually capable of doing and becoming'. These are Life, Bodily Health, Bodily Integrity, Senses, Imagination and Thought, Emotions, Practical Reason, Affiliation, Other Species, Play and Control over One's Environment. She asserts that developing these capabilities is concerned with ensuring quality of life. Furthermore she suggests that in the absence of any capability the individual would not have achieved a fully human existence. Gardner (1993) identifies seven 'intelligences', namely Linguistic, Logical-mathematical, Spatial, Musical, Bodily-kinesthetic, Interpersonal and Intrapersonal. He describes an intelligence as a biopsychological potential. All members of a species have the potential to exercise each of these intelligences.

These two categorisations of human potential arise from different perspectives on being human, but they share some common elements. Inherent in both are two factors, one being the identification of aspects or dimensions of humanness and the other being the identification of the expression of that dimension in some form of action. In both cases, in different ways, our embodiment is acknowledged as a fundamental human characteristic offering potential for development.

While physical literacy does not fit neatly into either Nussbaum's or Gardner's categorisations, there are a number of key features in the description of capabilities that lead to the categorisation of physical literacy as a capability rather than an intelligence. Nussbaum argues that each capability is valuable in itself and should not be seen as a means to other ends. She also explains that capabilities are cross-cultural and their development should be respected by all societies, governments and regimes. While she does not describe them as human rights she asserts that all human beings should be at liberty to exercise each capability and express themselves in ways that they choose. She talks of each capability as being an opportunity for functioning in a fully human way and argues that in nurturing the capability, each person should be treated as an end in themselves and not as a means to the ends of others. These features of a capability sit well alongside much that is explained in this text and, furthermore, are a reminder that at the heart of the debate is the well-being of every individual as a unique person worthy of respect. Finally, while Nussbaum does not support intrusive paternalism in developing these capabilities she advocates that attention should be paid to each in schooling.[1]

As we move through life we will each be confronted by different situations and contexts in relation to which our capabilities may need to be drawn on and adapted. The potential significance of each capability will not diminish as life is lived, although its expression may differ. This supports the assertion that physical literacy, described as a human capability, can be of value to every individual from cradle to grave. However, as Nussbaum indicates, it is open to each individual to capitalise on or disregard any aspect of their potential, and some people may choose not to develop or use a particular capability.

Premises that underpin the concept of physical literacy

The detailed consideration of some of the philosophical grounding of physical literacy is the subject of Chapter 3. However, at this stage it is useful to set down briefly some important premises that underpin the understanding of the concept. These premises are, in many ways, as challenging as adopting new terminology in respect of physical literacy itself. All have been alluded to in earlier sections of this chapter and are concerned with monism, different modes of our 'body' or embodiment and the interrelationships between human dimensions.

The first premise is that of our holistic nature. Physical literacy can only be conceptualised in the context of a monist approach to human beings. This attitude towards human life sees every individual as an indivisible whole. There is no sense in which we can talk about our embodiment or our 'body' as being a discrete aspect of our personhood. In line with recent scientific research as well as philosophical views, this designation is untenable. Physical literacy is a human capability expressed by an inherently embodied being; a being the nature of whom is characterised and delimited by an embodied presence in the world.

The second premise is based on an appreciation of the different modes through which the embodied dimension is lived. Physical literacy is founded on the acceptance that there is much more of significance to our embodied nature than just its object form. Alongside the 'body object' there is the 'body-as-lived' or lived embodiment. This latter mode of embodiment contributes to many aspects of life on a pre-reflective or pre-conscious level. However, the lack of conscious awareness of this mode of our embodiment, rather than making this dimension of ourselves less important, actually masks a great deal of its significance. It is interesting to note that the overall conscious awareness which human beings experience has been described as 'the tip of the iceberg' in the working of consciousness. It is proposed that the subconscious, functioning below our awareness, manages the majority of our everyday functioning. This is an example of monism in action. Without our conscious awareness, very many of our human dimensions are incorporated into our perceptions and actions. This is certainly the case with respect to our embodiment. As will be seen, embodied experiences play a significant part in, for example, perception, language development and interpersonal relationships. The term 'embodiment' is used throughout this book to signal reference to embodiment both as an instrument and as lived. Physical literacy is founded on and relies on an appreciation of embodiment in both modes.

The third premise which underpins the concept of physical literacy is that the development or deployment of any human dimension will, in almost every case, have an impact across all other dimensions. All aspects of an individual are irrevocably interrelated and interdependent. The exercise of any human dimension will affect all other dimensions. In line with this view, far from our embodied dimension being a somewhat separate aspect of our being, this mode of human expression operates in close collaboration with other modes. It will be seen that physical literacy can have significant effects on the development of, for example, cognition, imagination and reasoning. In a reciprocal fashion the development of potential with respect to other human dimensions can influence physical literacy. Enhancement of independence, creativity or intellectual abilities will all feed into nurturing physical literacy. Herein can be seen our holistic nature, the complexity of our make-up and the richness of human potential.

Physical literacy as defined in this text is founded on monism, the acceptance of different modes through which the embodiment is lived and the essential interdependent functioning of all dimensions of our human nature. This chapter has set out the definition of physical literacy, discussed the notion of physical literacy as a capability and highlighted the fundamental premises on which this capability is founded. Chapter 3 will look in detail at some of the philosophical thinking on which the concept is built.

Recommended reading

Gardner, H. (1993) *Frames of Mind: The Theory of Multiple Intelligences*. Fontana Press, London, Chs 1, 3, 4 and 9.

Nussbaum, M.C. (2000) *Women and Human Development: The Capabilities Approach*. Cambridge University Press, Cambridge, Ch. 1.

3 The philosophical underpinning of the concept of physical literacy

Margaret Whitehead

Introduction

This chapter looks at some aspects of the philosophical grounding of the concept of physical literacy. Two of the premises introduced in Chapter 2 will be subject to further explanation, these being monism and the contribution which the lived embodiment makes to many aspects of human existence. The latter discussion opens with an explanation of our nature as beings-in-the-world and this leads into an analysis of the role of the embodiment in perception and response.

The concept of physical literacy presented in this book has been developed over many years (Whitehead 1990). At root this study was initiated by a very strong commitment to the intrinsic value of embodied activity, a value that went beyond health and fitness and the refreshing benefits accrued for our mental capacities that are often achieved through a period of 'relaxing' physical activity. Early study of philosophy revealed a wide range of attitudes to our embodied dimension from those who dismissed 'it' as inferior to our mental capabilities to those that saw a key role for this aspect of human being. The latter, set out by philosophers who had no particular interest in or prejudice towards physical activity per se, opened up a completely new avenue of research. There was clearly potential, arising from the views of these philosophers, for the formulation of an argument that supported the value of the embodied dimension to every individual. This value would have real authority and be able to draw on the perceptions of and evidence from scholars. It seemed that, at last, those working in the field of movement, including physical educationists, would be able to identify the intrinsic value of their work. All practitioners with an interest in physical activity would be able to defend their area of expertise against the many who regard it as a recreational option rather than worthy of serious consideration. The outcome of this research has generated not merely a justification of physical activity throughout life, but a clear description of the significance of our embodied dimension from cradle to grave. It would be true to say that initial research has produced far more than had been hoped for or anticipated.

Monism

As a belief in monism is fundamental to the appreciation of the concept of physical literacy, some further clarification of this perspective on human existence is needed. The growing respect shown by some philosophers towards the embodied dimension rests on their commitment to the individual as a holistic being. A monist position rejects dualism with its contention that a person comprises two separable parts: the 'body' and the mind, with the 'body' viewed as an object and inferior to the mind. Furthermore, dualism sees little value in 'bodily' activity per se, other than sustaining existence and thereby prolonging the life of the mind. For many working in the field of physical activity this is not an acceptable position. We have experienced in ourselves and in others the profound and far-reaching effects of physical activity on many areas of human development. Designating our embodiment as purely an object or a machine is unacceptable and insensitive, disregarding and trivialising a key dimension of ourselves and one which, for many, is a highly significant aspect of the reality of life.

Monism, viewing the person as essentially an indivisible whole, would seem to align much more closely with the reality of human existence. This position is strongly advocated by many, for example, Ryle (1949), who worked to disprove the myth of the 'ghost in the machine', and Strawson (quoted in Gill 2000), who argued that the person is logically prior to any description of the dimensions from which the individual is comprised. In other words the person is first and foremost one entity and descriptions of different aspects of a person are isolating specific characteristics of human beings which, in fact, are not 'free-standing' but are part of an intricately integrated entity. There is not an issue of 'putting the separate parts together' as they are already functioning as a whole. It is regrettable that while there has been a clear lead from philosophers, as well as evidence from scientific research, both of which unequivocally support monism, the dualistic view of the human condition has remained firmly embedded in the Western psyche.

The roots of dualism can be traced back to Plato. Much of his philosophy rested on a view of the superiority of man's intellect as opposed to the inferiority of his 'body'. However, it was Descartes in the seventeenth century who was the most influential in establishing the notion of the two distinct characteristics of man – the mental and the physical, with the mental being inarguably the most significant. His justification for this view is based on his reasoning that the only thing he could not doubt was that he was thinking. Hence he asserted that 'I think therefore I am'. From his standpoint in history this view may be seen as uncontentious, if not obvious and logical.[1] The work of many recent writers, however, refutes this position and argues that we can only think because we are embodied.[2] For example, Bresler (2004: 36) expresses the interdependence of the mind and 'body' in proposing both that 'the body is in the mind' and that 'the mind is in the body'. These notions that the 'body is in the mind' and the 'mind is in the body' are very far from

Descartes' dualistic assertions. Interestingly, Modell (2006: 6) writes that 'with the famous exception of Eccles (1993) there are practically no neurobiologists who believe in a Cartesian dualism – the separation of matter from mind'.

Notwithstanding these assertions Descartes' views have become locked into the thinking of Western cultures to such an extent that habitual language use reaffirms dualism in the way it refers to the 'body' in terms of a noun – that is, as an object.[3] Individuals tend to talk about doing things 'to' the 'body' or 'with' the 'body'. Attention is frequently directed to our 'body object', for example, when we wash and clothe 'it', as we attempt to lose or gain weight and when we require attention from a doctor or other medical practitioner. Further attention is given to this 'concrete' dimension of ourselves in situations when 'its' instrumental powers are being called upon, such as when individuals want to open a jam jar, climb a ladder or play a game of tennis. This perspective on the 'body' is usually considered to be the extent of 'its' value.

What is overlooked in the language of dualism is the fact that there is more than one way in which the embodiment contributes to our nature as human beings. The experience of the lived embodiment – of living as the embodied beings we are – is seldom mentioned. More than this, it is the case that such a mode of living our embodiment appears inconceivable to many. And to say that you have not 'got' a 'body', but rather 'are' your 'body', is hard, if not impossible, for many people to understand and accept.

A significant challenge in establishing the concept of physical literacy is to help people understand the role of the lived embodiment and subsequently to show how this supports a monist view of human being. This will require a critical examination of people's almost unconscious presumption of dualism. Acceptance of the lived embodiment and of monism are crucial steps forward, as once our embodiment is appreciated as playing a fundamental role in existence, beyond 'its' obvious instrumental functions, the significance of this human dimension can be highlighted and can stand shoulder to shoulder alongside other human capabilities. The route to this understanding is, however, challenging, since it depends on coming to terms both with some of the tenets of existentialism, related to our nature as beings-in-the-world, and with a basic principle of phenomenology – that concerned with perception. These two areas of philosophy will now be explained.

Existentialism and phenomenology

Knowledge of some of the fundamental tenets of these schools of philosophy is essential to an understanding of physical literacy as set out in this text. While their titles are somewhat intimidating, the broad principles underlying their philosophical positions can be set out succinctly.

Fundamental to existentialist belief is that individuals create themselves as they live in and interact with the world. The persistent urge to interact with our surroundings is called 'intentionality'. Individuals are drawn, through intentionality, to perceive and to respond to everything and everyone around them. We live in a constant state of relating to the world, and thus our existence is played out as an ongoing dialogue between ourselves and our surroundings. This view is similar to the view that individuals are what they are, more via nurture than nature. Of course we arrive in the world with a wealth of potential capabilities, as well as inherited strengths and propensities – our nature, but what we make of ourselves depends on the experiences we have. At root individuals are 'beings-in-the-world'. A key principle underpinning existentialism is that 'existence precedes essence'. In other words our uniqueness, or essence, arises as a result of the experiences individuals have throughout life. Individuals do not come into the world 'ready-made'. We are as we are on account of the accumulation of all the situations in which we have been involved, whether by design or by chance.

The views of phenomenologists align well with those of existentialists. Phenomenologists are concerned to explain that every individual will perceive the world from the unique perspective of their previous experience. Individuals each 'make sense of the world' as it appears to them. As a corollary of this, each perception will modify our understanding of the world and in turn colour future perceptions. Each experience or perception will effect a change in ourselves, making us the unique person we are. Although it may be difficult to conceive, phenomenologists advocate that there is nothing hard and fast, nothing objective, 'out there' for us to understand, or come to know. What individuals perceive are 'phenomena', the word deriving from the Greek word 'appearances'. Phenomena are things as they appear to us, not necessarily things as explained by scientific enquiry.[4] Phenomena are the marriage of our previous experiences as they make sense of objects or situations in the environment. Familiar objects or situations will be imbued with previous connotations and their perception will be coloured by these connotations. A room in which we have previously had a difficult encounter will have very particular associations and thus will be perceived very differently from one for which it is our first visit. What individuals know of the outside world is achieved by the sense they make of it and this is the outcome of the sum total of our previous experiences. This aligns to what psychologists describe as assimilation. In assimilation the individual has to change or interpret what is perceived so that it is congruent with existing understanding. We 'see' things as they are for us. Although it is perhaps hard to envision, this means that, to a degree, everyone's world is different – unique to that individual. If I am allergic to wasp stings, the sight of a wasp will initiate immediate fear; if, however, I have had no previous alarming experiences with wasps their appearance will be either an irritant or of no consequence. It is interesting that psychologists link assimilation to accommodation, the latter describing the way in which the individual has to change in order to make sense of experience. To make sense of a situation, individuals may have to review previous ideas or perceptions to 'accommodate' new information. For example, the assessment of a person we have previously viewed as incompetent will have to change when we encounter that person carrying out a task with meticulous efficiency. There is, then, a two-way process. The perceiver 'reads' the world from their individual standpoint, colouring the situation in a way that enables them to 'make sense of it'. At the same time the individual may, to some extent, have to adapt, on account of what is perceived. In the need to accommodate new experiences, these novel experiences change the perceiver. Individuals both create their own world and are constantly changing, being ever modified by their interaction with the world.

In this way the link between existentialist and phenomenological views can be seen quite clearly. Phenomenologists explain why and how it is that, in existentialist terms, we are as we are, on account of the accumulated experiences we have had in effecting interaction with the world. As intentionality drives us to interact with our surroundings we change: knowledge, understanding and propensities are established, developed, modified, questioned and confirmed. Individuals become the persons they are at any one time.

From this starting point it can be reasoned that if individuals create themselves through interaction with the world, those human dimensions through which this interaction is made possible have a significant role to play in human experience and human existence. Interaction is effected through perception and response. It will be argued below that the embodied dimension, encompassing the embodiment-as-lived and the embodiment in its instrumental mode, has a key role to play in both aspects of interaction. It needs to be remembered that in the writings of some philosophers the role of embodiment in perception and response covers all sensory capacities, such as the ability to see and taste, as well as the response mechanisms involved in speech. However, in this text embodiment refers only to the embodied perceptual sense of proprioception and to response evidenced in gross and fine movement. Proprioception[5] provides the individual with a perceptual record of all interactions with the world that have been achieved through the deployment of the embodied dimension. This perceptual information is critical to understanding the world and contributes to the processes of both assimilation and accommodation.

The significant contribution of motility to both perception and response is in tune with the writings of existentialists and phenomenologists. There is no doubt that they are unequivocal about the key importance of our ability to move or motility. In fact in questioning their own views these philosophers repeatedly find themselves going back to our movement abilities as they ask 'how' and 'why' in relation to the nature of existence. As Gill (2000: 130) writes, '*Embodiment* is, after all, the axis or fulcrum of all tacit knowing, which in turn is the matrix of all explicit knowing.', and goes on to show how Polanyi (1966) was careful not to refer to the involvement of the motile capacities of our embodied dimension as a foundation but as the ongoing axis of thought and knowing. Our motile capability is seen as highly significant not least in that it is a very significant vehicle through which individuals can respond to the world and express themselves.

This section has set out the tenets of existentialism and phenomenology that lay the ground for an appreciation of the contribution of the embodied dimension to human existence. Further explanation is now needed in respect of the contribution of the embodiment to perception and response. Perception is the vehicle through which individuals come to understand the world, while response creates a living engagement with their surroundings.

Operative intentionality, embodied perception and response

As the previous section indicates, both existentialists and phenomenologists see humans as essentially beings-in-the-world who create themselves as they interact with their surroundings. Without this ongoing relationship with the world individuals would not realise the range of dimensions of which they are comprised or develop the capabilities that spring from these dimensions. Indeed, people would be without the experiences which provide the substance out of which they each become the individuals they are. This innate stimulus that individuals possess to be forever in an active relationship with the world is known as intentionality. Intentionality can be understood as our restless drive to perceive and respond to the world. The intentionality in which our embodiment plays the leading role is known as operative intentionality.

Operative intentionality may be understood as incorporating those aspects of perception and response in which the embodiment plays the key role. The role of our embodied dimension in perception arises from our experience of relating to an object or feature through movement. Our embodied interaction with an aspect in the world becomes an integral part of our understanding of that aspect. As we move in relation to an object or feature of the world, we experience a particular embodied relationship with that feature. This relationship then becomes integral to our understanding of that feature. In fact our perception of that feature incorporates the way we can relate to it effectively via our embodied dimension. Our perception of a flight of stairs incorporates the tacit knowledge of how to climb up and down these steps and our perception of a large jug of water incorporates the tacit knowledge of how we can lift this heavy object.

This aspect of perception is often overlooked on three counts. First, it operates at a pre-reflective level; that is, a level below consciousness, and is therefore overlooked and indeed taken for granted. Second, and as a consequence of this first situation, there is no descriptive language available to articulate this embodied relationship with the world. And finally this element of perception is almost imperceptively subsumed in the holistic grasp of an object afforded by human synaesthetic perception. Through synaesthesia the information from our different exteroceptors, such as eyes and ears, and from our interoceptors, such as those involved in proprioception, is automatically combined in such a way as to enable us to appreciate an object as a whole. Individuals do not have to piece together the different features of an object and combine these each time it is encountered. Within this understanding of an object or feature of the world, the operative element of perception is often disregarded. There is an irony in this. We are essentially beings in the world, beings who relate to the world via our embodiment. It is interesting to note that some writers talk about the 'knowing body', and Bresler (2004) entitles her book *Knowing Bodies, Moving Minds*. It is true to say that a great many aspects of the world are perceived by us from the perspective of our being embodied. This is endorsed by Merleau-Ponty (1964: 3) who explains that 'The perceiving mind is an incarnated mind'. He goes on to argue that in relation to operative intentionality there is an intimate relationship between perception and movement, and that these human dimensions are not separate from each other but function together.

Reflection on these insights reveals how the perception of things encompasses their significance to us as embodied beings. The final point to make about embodied perception concerns the similarities and differences in what we each perceive. Similarities will arise from the fact that individuals are all similarly embodied. Differences in perception will be the outcome of all previous experiences of that aspect of the world – the previous contexts in which individuals have encountered the feature and the situations in which this contact was made. Matthews (2006: 28) proposes that 'Our account of the world is given from our own point of view'. As was indicated earlier there is no 'one world', rather we each live in our own personal world; a place imbued with significances generated by our personal history of interactions.

Intentionality was described as incorporating both the urge to perceive and to respond to the world. As can be seen from the above outline of embodied perception, how individuals perceive or the sense they make of features in the world relates directly to ways in which they can deploy their embodied dimension in relating to these features. Within the context of operative intentionality it is therefore also impossible to separate perception from response. In fact there are two 'levels' at work in any response to the world. The most obvious 'level' is the conscious control of our embodied dimension as an instrument when we carry out a particular task, such as digging in the garden, writing someone's name or shooting in hockey. The other 'level' of response is perhaps harder to grasp, since it is effected by the lived embodiment below the level of consciousness. In respect of what might be called 'operative meaning' there is no language to describe the way in which, below the level of consciousness, our embodied dimension 'knows how to' interact with our surroundings. Polanyi (1966) refers to this as 'tacit' knowledge. Tacit knowledge is that which is acquired through interaction with the world but is not subject to conscious attention, it is learned through experience, rather than being articulated and subject to detailed description. It is generally related to 'know-how' and may be exemplified in the ability to ride a bicycle. The way in which individuals balance, steer and coordinate their embodied dimension is not 'known' in the way in which they know their address or the recipe to make a cake. Tacit knowledge is in a sense 'held' in our embodiment and called upon without conscious attention.[6] This 'knowledge' is described by Nietzsche (1969) as 'a great intelligence' that resides within our 'body'.[7]

In many cases where action is taken to interact with the environment there will be elements of conscious and unconscious initiation and control of our embodiment. In a sense the embodiment-as-instrument will be consciously controlled while the lived embodiment will draw from previous experience to provide the essential underpinning to our response to the world. Such is the adept use of this accumulated tacit knowledge that little attention is given to this embodied ability – it is presumed, passed by in silence and unappreciated. Much of this wealth of tacit knowledge will be acquired with little, if any, conscious attention as individuals learn to interact with the world. This learning is often carried out by trial and error, with much of it acquired as individuals develop the embodied competences that are usually associated with maturation such as walking, managing eating implements and dressing ourselves. The young child's restless exploration of, and experimentation with, features of the environment is a prime example of this learning. This is further exemplified in Chapter 9.

As may be seen from the above, our ability to respond depends to a great extent on our previous interactions with an object or feature. If we had never seen, touched, moved or used a chair before, we would look incredulously at this object, not knowing what we could or should do with it. Embodied interaction helps us to 'make sense' of our surroundings. This relationship is discussed further in Chapter 5 with respect to 'reading' the environment. The circle is unending; individuals perceive, use this information to respond and in responding add to the richness of their perception and to their bank of tacit embodied knowledge and repertoire of responses. In this cycle the individual changes, grows and develops.

This chapter has discussed monism and some of the tenets of existentialism and phenomenology as providing the foundation for the development of the concept of physical literacy. The concept relies on the acceptance of a monist approach with the embodiment playing a central role both as lived and in an instrumental role. The significant contribution of the lived embodiment in both perception and response has been outlined to demonstrate how our physical dimension, in this often forgotten mode, plays a significant part in human existence and in the development of each of us as a unique individual.

Recommended reading

Clark, A. (1997) *Being There: Putting Brain, Body and World Together Again.* MIT Press, London, Sections 3, 8 and Epilogue.

Gill, J. H. (2000) *The Tacit Mode.* State University of New York Press, New York, Chs 1, 2, 3, 5, 6.

Matthews, E. (2006) *Merleau-Ponty: A Guide for the Perplexed.* Continuum, London.

Whitehead, M.E. (1990) Meaningful existence, embodiment and physical education. *Journal of Philosophy of Education* 24, 1: 3–13.

4 Motivation and the significance of physical literacy for every individual

Margaret Whitehead

Introduction

This is the first of three chapters that will look in more detail at the attributes of physical literacy. This chapter will discuss the importance of motivation and the assertion that physical literacy enhances the quality of life. Consideration will then be given to the proposal that physical literacy is of significance and value to every individual and is achievable by all, whatever their age, embodied endowment and the culture within which they live.

The initial attribute (A and Aa) of physical literacy set out in Chapter 2 states that:

> *Physical literacy can be described as a disposition characterised by the motivation to capitalise on innate movement potential to make a significant contribution to the quality of life. All human beings exhibit this potential. However, its specific expression will depend upon individuals' endowment in respect of all capabilities, significantly their movement potential, and will be particular to the culture in which they live.*

Motivation and physical literacy

Motivation is understood to be a drive, a willingness and eagerness to take a particular action. At the heart of physical literacy is a desire to be active, to persist with an activity, to improve physical competence and to try new activities. Physically literate individuals will exhibit a 'joy of movement', and will celebrate, through movement, their ability to capitalise on their embodied capability. They will be confident in their physical abilities knowing that success is likely. A physically literate individual will enjoy a challenge, will be prepared to take time, expend effort and fund involvement in physical activity. Motivation is essential if there is to be the necessary application and concentration to thrive in the movement context, maintaining ability and making progress possible. A physically literate individual will have a positive attitude towards participation in physical activity and will take steps to be involved in this activity on a weekly or perhaps daily basis. Without this spur to action there will be little chance that physical literacy will be acquired or maintained.

It is suggested that the reason why many people seldom take part in physical activity is because of their lack of motivation. The term physical activity is used here to include such activities as walking and gardening, as well as all forms of sport, dance and other recognised pursuits such as skiing, pilates and bowling. It could be the case that earlier experiences, usually during schooling, have helped these individuals to develop their physical competence, but this experience has not resulted in their desire or interest in continuing with activity. This situation begs the question: Why do these people lack motivation?

It could be the case that aspects of their previous experience have been negative and this deters them from continuing to take part. Past experiences may not have been rewarding, with individuals experiencing little success. In the worst case scenarios they may have been subjected to humiliation, criticism and ridicule from significant others such as parents, teachers and peers. Individuals' confidence may have been damaged. Indeed, the thought of participating in physical activity may engender fear on the part of these non-participants. Establishing and sustaining physical literacy is highly dependent on experiences which individuals have encountered in respect of their involvement in physical activity. Chapter 7 considers the importance of nurturing self-respect if activity is to be maintained, while Chapter 14 looks at key pedagogical issues in the promotion of physical literacy. In brief, situations in which motivation is more likely to be promoted are those where appreciation is shown for effort and improvement, and thus self-confidence and self-esteem are enhanced. In these situations there is a celebration of each individual's abilities and mutual respect is shown between all those involved. Motivation essentially arises from the confidence and self-esteem acquired through experience; that is, experience which has been perceived as successful and has been recognised as such.

Motivation to be involved in all forms of embodied activity is innate in the young child, being the expression of operative intentionality to engage with the world. A discussion of movement and the young child can be found in Chapter 9. There seems to be a drive, a need, an insatiable curiosity to explore and interact with every aspect of the environment. This is the purest example of being-in-the world and living through or creating the self, through interaction with the world. The young child seems to be in a constant state of dissonance, urgently needing to find equilibrium. This is an early form of intrinsic motivation and is characteristically played out predominantly in movement. The ideal scenario is one in which the child's natural motivation to explore and experiment with ways of interacting with the environment is never lost. The individual continues to enjoy physical activity for its own sake, reaping the wide range of benefits this brings to the enrichment of life.

It is sad that this intrinsic motivation can be lost on account of less than positive experiences that young people encounter. Intrinsic motivation can be described as a drive to take action for the benefit of the experience itself and not as a means to other ends. In situations where motivation has been lost, measures have to be taken to encourage these younger or older people to re-engage in physical activity and experience the positive outcomes of participation. Examples of individuals returning to being physically active can be found in Chapters 8 and 10. Forms of extrinsic motivation may be needed to initiate a return to being active. Typically this motivation takes the form of approval and praise from another person or some form of reward such as a treat for a young person or the possibility of losing weight for an adult. The goal with these individuals would be to offer opportunities for success, to nurture interest, and to re-ignite a drive to capitalise on physical potential. Where this is successful there can be a return to intrinsic motivation, with individuals becoming self-motivated and no longer reliant on others to spur them into action. In other words, individuals acquire a positive disposition to participate in physical activity and thus become physically literate.

Physical literacy as enhancing quality of life

It is proposed that being physically literate can make a significant contribution to the quality of life. As has been outlined in Chapter 3, our nature as beings-in-the-world who create themselves from interaction with the environment, means that all aspects of our being that afford this contact are highly significant. The wider, richer and more acute our perception of, and interplay with, our surroundings the more we will come to know the world and realise our potential. The only way individuals can achieve their full potential, open up the many avenues of development and live a fulfilled life is to actively engage with the environment. As the embodied dimension is implicated in much of this interaction there is no doubt that this human capability has the potential to play a central role in enhancing the quality of life. The role of this dimension in perception and response was outlined in Chapter 3. However, what was perhaps not stressed was the way in which this mode of interaction permeates nearly everything we do in life. Indeed, our embodied capability is so integral to life that it is all but impossible to conceive of an unembodied existence. It might be true to say that without our motile embodied capability there would be no existence. Supporting this perspective, Merleau-Ponty (1962: 166) describes existence as 'perpetual incarnation', and Sartre (1957: 476) writes, 'for human reality, to be is to act'.

This situation reveals the fundamental importance of our embodied dimension and hence physical literacy in life as we know it. There are at least two ways in which our embodied capability makes a significant contribution to life. Both of these ways develop from our nature as a single indivisible entity, in which experiences are all-pervading, affecting, informing and changing us as people. The broader contribution in relation to the realisation of a fuller life will be looked at first, followed by a consideration of some more specific contributions to our flourishing, being in respect of the development of other human characteristics such as cognition and language.

Physical literacy, as the expression of a fundamental capability, is one vehicle through which individuals can realise and develop their characteristic human nature. A number of writers talk about our becoming more human as we exercise any of our potential capabilities. There is a sense in which these experiences are self-affirming, intrinsically satisfying and rewarding. Each capability is of value in its own right and will enable the individual to blossom in a particular way. However, each will also contribute to the well-being of the whole person. For example, exercising our powers to sing, appreciate art masterpieces or grapple with mathematical formulae has its own positive feedback to our personal fulfilment and sense of self. Each of these activities will make us who we are and build our self-confidence. Physical literacy is no exception.

Capitalising on embodied potential can undoubtedly contribute to the sense of self. The self-respect and self-confidence acquired through the deployment of embodied potential can be profoundly fulfilling. Using this human capability brings to the fore an essential and fundamental aspect of our being. Through exercise and challenge of the powers of the embodied dimension, individuals celebrate a unique aspect of humanness. More than this we celebrate the roots of our being, the wellspring of many of the other capabilities. Effective deployment of the embodied capability is a holistic and rewarding experience. While achievement will be relative to the person in question, the experience of growing competence will be of a similar nature. This could be realised in carrying out a simple skill for the first time, learning to use a novel gadget, taking part in a new sport or mastering a highly complex move in gymnastics or diving. There is undoubtedly potential for intrinsic satisfaction in the deployment of this human capability. This can be a self-affirming experience of ourselves as embodied beings; a satisfying and profound experience of improving physical competence, of growing independence and of self-realisation.

In addition to this intrinsically valuable and satisfying experience of involvement in physical activity available to all, which is often overlooked, there are, of course, a number of what might be called additional benefits of deploying the embodied dimension. There are a range of well-documented health benefits such as preventing obesity, building up resistance to certain forms of cancer and maintaining joint flexibility. In addition, there may be the invigoration brought about by exercise in the fresh air, with the beneficial physiological effects of stimulating the cardiovascular system, not least through the secretion of body chemicals such as endorphins that both relax and energise the state of being. There may be the refreshing experience of simply having the freedom to move after hours of seated work; the pleasure brought about by calling on a different human capability. There may also be a sense of belonging in a group activity setting, with the enjoyment of sharing a common interest with others, and the positive experience of being valued and respected by other people. Physical activity can also have beneficial effects to allay stress and contribute therapeutically to the recovery from a range of health and well-being problems.

Beyond the self-affirming and additional benefits that arise from deploying, developing and sustaining physical competence there is growing support for the way in which capitalising on the potential of the embodied dimension can contribute to other human capabilities such as cognition, language, reasoning and the expression of emotions. This position, championed by Merleau-Ponty and now endorsed by a range of current philosophers and scientists, is founded on the monist belief in the indivisibility or interdependence of the 'mind' and the 'body'. Lakoff and Johnson explain (1999: 3) that 'The mind is inherently embodied'. Burkitt (1999) elaborates on this and writes:

> [W]hat we call 'mind' only exists because we have bodies that give us the potential to be active and animate within the world, exploring, touching, seeing, hearing, wondering, explaining; and we can only become persons and selves because we are located bodily at a particular place in space and time, in relation to other people and things around us.
>
> (Burkitt 1999: 12)

This view turns on its head the notion that our 'mental' faculties are separate from, independent of and somehow far superior to our embodied capacities. Sheets-Johnstone (1992: 43) also challenges this view squarely by asserting that 'A human intelligence bereft of a body would be an intellectual cripple'. There is no doubt of the significant role that the intellect plays in the way individuals live their lives, and no one can argue with this, but what is so striking is the way that, repeatedly, writers refer back to our embodiment as the wellspring of the intellect.

While there is no doubt that the contribution of our embodied capacities is of significance throughout life, or as Polanyi explains, as detailed in Gill (2000), is the 'ongoing axis' of thought and knowing, our embodied interaction with our surroundings in the early days, months and years of life are particularly critical, and much has been written about the way in which our embodied dimension is involved in how a child develops.

For example, Clark (1997) suggests that cognitive development cannot be understood in isolation from children's intimate relationships with the world via their embodied dimension. Similarly, Sheets-Johnstone (2002) describes infants as 'apprenticed' to their embodied dimension. From birth, the child is actively perceiving and responding, becoming familiar with such features as heat and cold, texture, near and far, weight and spatial relationships of 'on top of' and 'underneath', to name but a few areas of basic knowledge. The lack of speech in the first eighteen months or so of life should not be taken to mean that no learning is taking place. A great deal of learning is occurring, in respect of developing physical competence, in relation to making sense of the world around, and in the early formulation of concepts that are the foundation of cognition. Many writers concur that there is no sense that our embodied capacities are secondary to any of our other capabilities; rather, the opposite is the case. In fact scientists are now beginning to show that it is through the embodied dimension that many of the other capabilities are able to develop. The nurturing of physical competence ensures that a framework that is essential to many aspects of development is in place. For example, it is suggested that it is from the foundation of coming to understand the world through embodied interaction that the young child begins to attribute meaning via language. The meaning referred to goes beyond the often first achievement of 'naming' people and things. Children develop the ability to appreciate, and thus name, characteristics such as weight, size and shape. They can identify spatial relationships such as under and over, near and far, as well as aspects of time – now, soon, later, tomorrow. All these linguistic concepts arise from the embodied experience of the environment.

Burkitt (1999) argues that perception and embodied action form the basis of meaning. Meaning is, therefore, not created as a result of applying the rules of cognition or the rules of grammatical correctness but arises through our embodied interaction with the world. Other writers support this view, explaining that propositional knowledge only becomes comprehensible in the context of embodied experience, and that the concepts individuals develop should not be viewed as the sole purview of a disembodied innate faculty of mind. There is no such thing as a disembodied mind. What individuals know, what is 'in our mind' is as a direct result of our embodied interaction with the world.[1]

Lakoff and Johnson (1999) develop this line of thought further and show how a grasp of basic concepts forms the ground for rationality and reasoning. Typical of their assertions is that 'Reason is not disembodied . . . but arises from the nature of our brains, bodies, and bodily experience' (1999: 4). For example, they attribute a clear embodied basis to the 'weighing' of one idea against another and of the 'balancing' of one potential outcome against another. Concepts such as these are experienced initially pre-reflectively via embodied interaction with the world; however, these interactions provide the fundamental understanding of difference and differential outcomes. Sheets-Johnstone (2002: 104) reiterates this view in asserting that 'rationality is first and foremost a bodily logos'. She explains that the basis of rationality is 'sense-making' and that the acquisition of this capability depends wholly on the nature of the embodiment.

As well as the embodied dimension being critical in the development of areas of cognition such as concept formulation, language and reasoning, a number of writers see a clear role for this human dimension in respect of emotion. In looking very briefly at this view, two issues will be mentioned, namely the importance of the emotions and the involvement of the embodied dimension in the experience and presentation of emotions. In respect to the importance of the emotions there seems no doubt that they are a fundamental aspect of human life. There is a great deal written about this aspect of our human nature. For example, authors such as McMurray and Dunlop refer to emotions as of central importance in human life – indeed, as the core or essence of life as we know it. In fact McMurray (1935, quoted in Dunlop 1984) asserts that the intellect arises from our emotional life: 'is rooted in it, draws its nourishment and sustenance from it'. The emotions are not simply one element of life but are an integral and essential part of being human.

Considering the involvement of the embodied dimension in emotion it is essential to move away from a position that sees emotions as a discrete aspect of human functioning. In fact there is no such thing as a 'disembodied emotion'. It is not the case that what individuals perceive, or perhaps better, what individuals see and hear, of another's behaviour is merely the 'outward display' of an 'inner state' or emotion. Best (1974) supports this and explains that the emotion is in the movement itself. Our embodied dimension is not a passive vehicle for expressing an emotion. Movement or actions are the very material of emotion. Movement does not reveal an emotion; it is part and parcel of the emotion. Burkitt (1999: 116) expresses the view that 'the physical component of an emotion is vital to our experience of it', and goes on to argue that embodied involvement in the experience of emotion is not the outcome of a mental state but an integral part of the emotion itself. He further explains that emotions arise from our interaction with others and our response to situations in which we find ourselves. Emotions have an essential relational element and are part of the human communication system. As such they are important to sensitive interaction with others. In perceiving others we need to be alert to and empathetic with the emotion being expressed. While there are basic emotions which all human beings share, the specific expression of emotion is regulated by the accepted practices in a social class or culture. As Burkitt explains (1999: 124): 'emotional feeling is at one and the same moment, produced and regulated'. Our embodied dimension is integral to the expression of emotion and is also involved in the control of the emotion, ensuring that this is culturally appropriate and socially acceptable.[2]

In the light of the views that the embodied dimension is an essential component in emotional experience and expression, as well as playing a part in the regulation of emotion and in communicating with others, it could be argued that a sensitive awareness of the embodied dimension is valuable to this aspect of human life. Physically literate individuals endowed with versatility, confidence and competence with respect to their embodied dimension would seem to be in a better position to experience, express and appreciate different emotions, and also to monitor and control emotions to conform with cultural expectations. This issue will be returned to in Chapter 6. This section of the chapter has looked at the way in which developing our embodied capability can enhance other aspects of our human nature. Gallagher (2005: 247) sums up this position:

> [N]othing about human experience remains untouched by human embodiment: from the basic perceptual and emotional processes that are already at work in infancy, to a sophisticated interaction with other people; from the acquisition and creative use of language, to higher cognitive faculties.

Physical literacy as achievable by all

This area of discussion relates to the element in the definition of physical literacy that claims it is a universal concept (see also Whitehead 2007d). It is proposed that all human beings have the potential to realise this capability, notwithstanding the fact that its expression will be particular to the potentials with which the individual is endowed and the culture within which they live. There are, therefore, two main areas to consider. The first relates to an individual's embodied potential and the second to cultural context.

Our embodied dimension is a significant and indeed essential human asset. As embodied beings, we all, in a sense, 'live through' our embodied dimension. Embodied interaction with our surroundings is the ground of our development, including knowledge of the world, self-awareness and self-confidence. This view was one of the key insights of existentialists and phenomenologists with their description of the human condition as essentially embodied in-the-world. On these grounds it is argued strongly that physical literacy is applicable to all, whatever the nature of their embodied endowment. Everyone can accrue great benefit from being physically literate, that is from developing their embodied interaction with the world.

The issue concerning whether the capability of physical literacy is attainable by all or is achievable only by the 'physically gifted' has attracted considerable debate. It is argued in this text that physical literacy is within the scope of every individual, whatever their embodied potential, but that the expression of this human capability will differ in respect of the individual's embodied endowment. It is regrettable that this is seen as an area for debate, somehow discounting the potential of many people and discouraging them from developing this aspect of their humanness. That this point needs to be brought to the fore would seem to shed some light on the way embodied abilities are viewed in Western culture. There appears to be an all too readily adopted attitude in Western culture of self-deprecation in respect of the way individuals regard their embodied capability. Many people dismiss suggestions that they have any potential in this area. They purposefully avoid any involvement in physical activity, asserting that they have no ability and 'it is not for them'. It may be the case that the media are partly to blame for the development of this unfortunate attitude. Television and the press focus on high-level performance and international competition, they champion sports stars, show and describe amazing physical feats and give time and space to the development of extreme sports. The relentless exposure to high-level performance in Western media, with its hidden message that this is the only manifestation of embodied ability worthy of attention, results in many people judging themselves to be 'physically incompetent'. As the level of performance 'on show' is out of their reach, many seem to conclude that physical activity is 'not for them'. They say 'I am no good at sport'. They are not motivated to take part in any physical activity and are lacking in confidence, anticipating failure, embarrassment and loss of self-esteem. The deployment of their capability in respect of their embodied dimension is not perceived as a potential source of achievement, of satisfaction or of a feeling of well-being. This is very sad and should not be the case.

Indeed this is not the case – almost without exception all have the potential to achieve physical literacy and benefit from its expression. Apart from the very severely physically disabled, all individuals possess the building blocks of physical literacy. As such these competences are available for us all to use and develop, beyond the essential embodied involvement with the world that is integral to life in general. Opportunities for capitalising on our embodied capability through some form of structured physical activity are many and various – both in the nature of the activity and the degree of the challenge. It must surely be the case that each one of us can find a context or contexts within which we can experience satisfaction and reward in expressing and developing physical literacy. Each individual will be on their own personal physical literacy journey. All can make progress, and each will display physical literacy in the context of their endowment. The important element is that individuals are making progress on their own personal journey. The benefits of physical literacy are available to everyone.

Physical literacy, disability and the older adult population

In the context of the claim that physical literacy is a universal concept the question it is often raised as to how applicable or achievable this capability is to those who have what might be broadly described as, 'a disability'. The problem arises, in part, from the aforementioned preoccupation with high-level skilful performance as being the principal goal in participation in physical activity. The value and indeed relevance of physical activity for those with a disability is often doubted, with perhaps only the physical fitness or therapeutic aspects being felt to be worthwhile. However, parents, carers and teachers of these individuals need to appreciate that any development in physical competence is valuable and comparisons with those who have no disability are out of place.

Reference to attitudes to learning to read may be useful here. Interestingly there are what is known as 'reading ages'. Whatever 'reading age' is attained the individual is said to be able to read. The ability to read, even at a very basic level, is recognised as an achievement and valued in respect of the opportunities this affords to the individual. The more competent individuals are at reading the more potential there is for them to widen their horizons and enrich their lives. In the same way when individuals take even a small step on their physical literacy journey, this is valuable and should be celebrated. All individuals should be encouraged to make progress, thus widening their horizons and enriching their life options. The focus on achievement for those with a disability is not relative to others, but is expressed in the charting of progress on the personal physical literacy journey of each person.

Individuals with a disability may be at the start of their journey in becoming physically literate and they may be travelling very slowly; however, their progress will be as significant as the refinement of a higher order embodied capacity for those who have already travelled some way. I would argue strongly that any progress in respect of physical literacy, from whatever starting point, will have a profound impact on the individual concerned. This applies equally to the challenge of climbing stairs, managing a knife and fork or catching a ball for a disabled youngster, to the achievement of the necessary coordination to drive a car, to keeping a rally going in tennis, or to scaling a particularly challenging cliff face for those who have no difficulties. Each individual has the potential to be physically literate but the expression of this capacity will be as unique to the individual as their particular personality. Movement work with those with a disability will be discussed further in Chapter 11; however, there is no doubt that every individual can benefit enormously from developing their physical literacy. Growth in coordination or a small step in coming to grips with a physical task can be tremendously rewarding for those with difficulties, giving them added self-esteem, self-confidence and ultimately greater independence.

Another closely related issue concerns the value of physical literacy and its attainment in the case of the older adult population. There is a commonly held view that when an individual reaches old age physical activities are irrelevant – these activities are for the 'young and fit'. However, this is profoundly untrue, as will be exemplified in Chapter 10. There is growing evidence that nurturing movement competence throughout the later stages of the lifecourse adds hugely to the quality of life of older people. It is not so much developing an individual's embodied potential, as with younger people, but rather to do with maintaining physical activity options and thus enhancing the confidence, independence and self-respect of these members of society.

As with any human potential, there is a positive experience associated with exercising a capability, and indeed with any progress, however small the step. What is being advocated here is the nurturing of a positive attitude towards one's embodied potential and to the realisation that physical activity is innately rewarding and self-affirming. The motivation, confidence and competence to take part in physical activity is within the grasp of us all. What are most worrying are situations where individuals go out of their way to avoid all physical activity, be this house cleaning, walking, throwing or kicking a ball or swimming. Once there is the preparedness to take part in physical activity, to give time and expend effort, then physical literacy can be a personal asset and play a part in enriching life.

Physical literacy and culture

A second area of debate in respect of the universality of the concept of physical literacy relates to the relevance and significance of the capability to the socio-cultural context in which an individual lives. There are, perhaps, three issues to consider. One relates to the fact that all individuals share the same embodied structure and functioning, irrespective of the culture of which they are a part, and another concerns the physical demands that the lifestyle within a culture may make on our embodied dimension. The final issue relates to attitudes to the embodied dimension that are prevalent in a particular culture.

With respect to the first issue it would be argued that, as human beingss, whenever and wherever life is lived, the embodied capability is a significant aspect of being human. Existentialists and phenomenologists would not think twice about the validity of this proposition. Two fundamental aspects of our human situation that were discussed in the previous section are pertinent here. First, that human life is lived, necessarily, from an embodied standpoint, with all knowledge of the world and all development of the individual deriving from embodied interaction with our environment. Second, the significant role played by our embodied dimension in the development of other aspects of human functioning such as cognition, the formation of concepts and reason. Gibbs (2006: 41) endorses this by writing 'perception, cognition and language are thoroughly embodied.' This position is supported by contemporary writers such as Sheets-Johnstone (1994) and Nussbaum (2000). The former, while accepting the influence of culture on our movement patterns and behaviour, is always quick to remind us of our roots as embodied animate beings, who share a common parentage through evolution. While Nussbaum identifies a number of 'Central Human Functional Capabilities' that pertain to every individual irrespective of their cultural context, she argues (2000: 73) that all these capabilities need to be nurtured if individuals are to achieve what Marx called being 'truly human'. Among her named capabilities she cites a range of aspects related to our embodied nature. There is considerable support for the view that deploying our embodied capability is fundamental to life as a human being, whenever and wherever life is lived. On these grounds the concept of physical literacy can be seen as universally relevant.

The second issue relates to the expression of physical literacy in the context of the different physical demands that a culture may make on the human embodied dimension. This can be looked at on two levels. At a fundamental level it is proposed that being similarly embodied, the range of movement patterns and movement capacities outlined in Chapters 5 and 15 are common to all human beings. While it may be observed that the range of movement components identified has a 'Western cultural' flavour, the reader is challenged to rewrite these for the hunter-gatherer, the crofter and the nomadic Inuits. It is doubtful that many would be deleted, although the use and expression of some may vary. The basic components of physical competence will therefore be the same in any culture. That having been said, on a contingent level, different cultures will make different demands on our physical literacy and provide different opportunities for challenging this human capability. For example, in Western culture in everyday life individuals are seldom expected to walk far, carry heavy loads or get involved in physically taxing tasks such as digging. While there are still some areas or work, such as those in the building trades that require heavy manual labour, the nature of most of the tasks that are necessary today require more intricate coordination, more precision and less use of large muscle groups.[3] For example, individuals need to be able to drive a car and operate a computer. It would be interesting to look at the particular demands on the embodied dimension of those living in medieval times and those currently living in the third world. It would seem to be the case that all human beings will call upon their fundamental movement competences, but certain of these will be drawn on more often and become more highly developed to reflect the demands of a specific lifestyle.

There will also be differences in the structured physical activities that are available. Every culture has its specific forms of physical activity, be they dance genres, types of swimming or competitive sports. These activities will, in a sense, be part of the fabric of a society and may feature in education in order to initiate the young into accepted forms of cultural activity. In Western culture one might cite competitive team games and athletics, while in some Eastern cultures initiation in education might be into martial arts and forms of dance. While the fundamentals of physical literacy will be essentially the same for all, the way they are deployed will vary according to the parent culture.

Burkitt (1999) would concur with this and argues that while the embodied dimension and therefore, in our terms, physical literacy, plays a key role in the life of all human beings, the specific role of the embodiment differs markedly depending on the culture within which individuals live. He writes (1999: 25):

> However, as far as human beings are concerned, it is not just the interaction between organism and environment that defines our being, for these 'movements' of life are also interrelated with, and affected by, our history as social and cultural groups.

Included here are not only the more functional aspects of deploying our embodied dimension but also the demands made by operating effectively in the context of established social practices, including the particular form of interpersonal relationships that are seen to be acceptable in a culture.

The final aspect to be considered follows from the suggestion above, and concerns the specific way in which the embodied dimension is viewed by a particular culture. Gibbs (2006) discusses this issue and observes, interestingly, that human beings inhabit 'physical environments imbued with culture' (2006: 36) and that our embodied dimension itself incorporates 'cultural meanings and memories' (2006: 37). He goes on to discuss how many of our embodied experiences are rooted in the social-cultural context in which individuals live. There is a sense that our embodied dimension has particular 'meaning' that incorporates established cultural attitudes. He concludes by saying: 'Rather than being a biological given, embodiment is a category of social analysis, often revealing complex dimensions of interactions' with other humans and the environment. A great deal has been written about attitudes to the embodied dimension both throughout the history of man and in different cultures. This is a fascinating area with implications to the expression of physical literacy, but is beyond the scope of this book.[4] Cultural issues are referred to again in Chapter 12.

It is essential here, however, to signpost the implications for physical literacy of the way our embodied dimension is viewed in what Shilling (2003) refers to as high modernity in developed Western cultures. As is ably described by Shilling (2003) and Grogan (2008) in their texts on the sociology of the body, there is a worrying trend for people not only to perceive themselves predominantly in terms of their embodiment-as-object, but also to judge themselves based on the attitudes of others to this aspect of their personhood. Society, through its members, exerts huge pressure on people in respect of the 'ideal body' – how they should look and present themselves. The media play a significant part in this process. The power of the media is picked up again in Chapter 8. A very unfortunate outcome of this is that individuals forget there is more to themselves than their embodiment-as-object. Self-esteem is damaged when they perceive they do not match up to the ideal model and in some cases they feel alienated from their embodiment-as-object. Girls and women are most at risk here (see also Whitehead 2007b, 2007c). It is suggested that Western society should be far more accepting of variations in the size and shape of the embodied dimension and should work to develop positive attitudes in respect of the physical competence of the many rather than the few. Involvement in physical activity, where sensitively handled, can enhance attitudes to individuals' embodiment and hence to their self-respect, self-confidence and quality of life.

This chapter has looked in more detail at the importance of motivation in the maintenance of physical literacy and the issue of universal applicability of the concept. It has been argued that physical literacy is achievable by all, including those with a disability and the older adult population. Each individual is on their own personal physical literacy journey. With respect to physical literacy in different cultures, it has been argued that as human beings we all share this capability; however, its specific expression will always be influenced by the particular demands and opportunities evident within a society, and by the cultural significance of this dimension of ourselves. The next chapter looks at physical competence and the attribute of physical literacy related to effective interaction with a wide range of physical environments.

Recommended reading

Burkitt, I. (1999) *Bodies of Thought: Embodiment, Identity and Modernity*. Sage, London.

Clark, A. (1997) *Being There: Putting Brain, Body and World Together Again*. MIT Press, London, Sections 1, 2, 3, 4, 5, 8 and Epilogue.

Gibbs, R.G. Jr. (2006) *Embodiment and Cognitive Science*. Cambridge University Press, Cambridge, Ch. 2.

Lakoff, G. and Johnson, M. (1999) *Philosophy in the Flesh: The Embodied Mind and its Challenge to Western Thought*. Perseus Books Group, Basic Books, New York, Chs 1, 3, 4 and 5.

Whitehead, M.E. (2007a) Physical literacy and its importance to every individual. Paper given at the National Disability Association of Ireland, Dublin, January.

5 Physical literacy, physical competence and interaction with the environment

Margaret Whitehead

Introduction

This chapter will discuss the second and third attributes of a physically literate individual. Physical competence and physically challenging situations will be considered first. This will be followed by an explanation of the notion of 'reading' the physical environment in the context of the philosophical standpoint that describes humans as essentially beings-in-the-world.

The second and third attributes (B and C) of physical literacy set out in Chapter 2 state that:

> *Individuals who are physically literate will move with poise, economy and confidence in a wide variety of physically challenging situations.*

> *Physically literate individuals will be perceptive in 'reading' all aspects of the physical environment, anticipating movement needs or possibilities and responding appropriately to these with intelligence and imagination.*

Physical literacy and physical competence

While physical competence is a central attribute displayed by a physically literate individual, it must be remembered that this attribute alone can never be the sole constituent of physical literacy. Expression of physical competence must be accompanied by a positive attitude towards activity. Physically literate individuals are not only competent but also confident in respect of the movement potential with which they have been endowed. They are motivated to capitalise on their embodied dimension. Notwithstanding these cautionary comments, the nature of human movement as the basis of physical competence needs to be clarified. The elements of physical competence set out below can be seen to provide a description of the nature of the journey each individual will be taking in respect of physical literacy. The goal is to make progress, not to master every aspect of movement competence.

Over the years a number of systems of analysis have been proposed in respect of human movement. These have spelled out the constituents of movement and the ways in which these components can be combined in the production of sophisticated skills and techniques. The analysis outlined below and detailed further in Chapters 9 and 15 in no way claims to be the definitive method of describing human movement. However, it springs from the knowledge and experience of a number of movement specialists. The analysis incorporates elements of other approaches to this task, all of which have valuable contributions to make to understanding the nature of movement, its building blocks and the complexities of combining these constituents. Understanding the nature of human movement is essential to appreciate both the range of movements possible and the ways in which movement can be made more efficient and effective. Each analysis sets out the material that can be covered in the movement field, providing a vocabulary and a language that can be used to describe movement. Those concerned to promote physical competence need to be able to use movement language fluently both in planning and in working with participants. A grasp of the constituents of human movement is a fundamental tool for all those concerned to nurture physical literacy.

The analysis outlined below is designed to embrace movement from birth, through to the very specific movement patterns evident in discrete activity contexts such as a competitive game, mountaineering or contemporary dance. The analysis comprises four aspects of movement that recognise a growing refinement of deploying embodied capability. These are:

- a young child's movement vocabulary
- movement capacities
- movement patterns – general and refined
- specific movement patterns that are contextually designed for a particular activity setting.

A young child's movement vocabulary is founded on the physical compe-tences normally exhibited as the physical growth and development of the newborn child proceeds through the first few years of life. This vocabulary encompasses movements such as rolling, crawling, walking, grasping, lifting, waving and clapping. Through continued use this first movement vocabulary becomes established in the movement memory. The quality of executing this vocabulary is enhanced by its repeated application in a variety of situations. This stage in developing physical competence is explained further in Chapter 9.

Refinement of the young child's vocabulary and indeed of this vocabulary throughout life is achieved through acquiring and applying a range of movement capacities to these basic competences. These are described as follows:

- simple, such as balance, coordination and flexibility;
- combined, for example, poise, which requires balance and core stability, and agility, which combines flexibility, balance and coordination;

- complex, involving further combinations of capacities; for example, hand–eye coordination needing orientation in space, agility and dexterity.

While capacities are generally developed from simple through combined to complex there is no built-in hierarchy in the order in which capacities from each category are incorporated into the young child's vocabulary. The development of movement competence is more like exploring a wide terrain rather than following a narrow path up a mountain.

The next aspect in this movement analysis is the development of general and refined movement patterns. The constituents of the young child's movement vocabulary are progressively streamlined as capacities are applied to what might be called innate or general movement patterns. General patterns would include striking, while refined patterns would include the development of striking as batting. As a final stage, development of specific movement patterns produces contextually designed patterns that are called for in particular activity settings. The specific pattern of batting evolves into the batting technique required in cricket or baseball. As can be seen, the analysis suggests that movement comprises movement patterns arising through growth and maturation from birth and then honed through the application of movement capacities into ever more sophisticated techniques. Further clarification of this progressive refinement is found in Chapter 15.

It is useful to remember that while the above analysis has focused on physical competence in the field of structured physical activity, movement patterns and movement capacities are constantly being called on in everyday life. For example, walking, running, lifting and carrying are everyday activities, as are writing, using a knife and fork, and keyboard skills. Individuals' employment may also demand the use of specific patterns and capacities. A chef, a hairdresser and a decorator will each use a particular range of movement patterns in their work. Each movement pattern will rely on capacities such as control, coordination and flexibility, and each pattern will become more refined with use. Physical competence, alongside other attributes of physical literacy, is evident and indeed of value beyond structured physical activity settings into life as a whole.

There are two observations to be made in respect of the range of movement competences described above.

The first observation concerns the breadth and depth of the potential of the embodied dimension in relation to physical literacy. As indicated above and developed in later chapters, individuals are capable of enacting a wide range of movement patterns and of refining these through the incorporation of numerous capacities. It is suggested that the fostering of physical literacy is best grounded in the nurturing of a wide range of a young child's potential movement vocabulary, the development of all the movement capacities and the application of these capacities in the effective performance of as many general movement patterns as possible. From this foundation a range of specific and contextualized movement patterns can be developed. As will be discussed in Chapter 15, this grounding will enable individuals to select one or more activity context which both matches their movement strengths and offers experiences that fulfil their personal interests. Furthermore, as adulthood and older age are reached and embodied potential and personal interests change, individuals will be able to capitalise on earlier experience and find satisfaction in different activity settings. This recommendation has implications for planned movement opportunities for children and adolescents. A broad experience of movement patterns and activity settings is important, as this will enable individuals to establish sound physical competence, as appropriate to their endowment, and provide each with a range of experiences from which they can select activity contexts in which to participate. The key here is breadth and balance of experience. This pertains to whatever system of movement analysis is used. A broad base of physical competence is essential, as this constitutes the foundation of physical literacy. As the concept has been developed, questions have been asked in respect of whether an individual who specialises in and is outstanding at one activity context, possibly at the expense of taking part in any other form of movement activity, can be said to be physically literate. There is much to debate here. In the worst case scenario high-performing athletes may hone their movement patterns and consequently their physique to such an extent that participation in other activities becomes problematic. Perhaps an example here is a professional weight lifter. In another scenario a high-performing athlete may continue to take part in a range of other movement activities, any of which could be taken up as and when opportunities arise. There would be a case to describe the second athlete, but not the first, as physically literate. It is probably the case that overspecialisation can be at the expense of physical literacy and, far from opening doors in respect of lifelong participation, may, in fact, close them.

The second observation picks up the points made at the end of Chapter 4 concerning the expression of physical literacy in different cultures. It was suggested that while the constituents of physical competence are common to everyone, all being similarly embodied, their development and refinement will, to some extent, be culturally defined. Differences in the deployment of this competence and thus in the expression of physical literacy will reflect both the demands and expectations in everyday life and the forms of structured physical activity that are characteristic of the country or region. However, this does not change the need to nurture a wide range of young children's movement vocabulary and to help them develop movement capacities. The selection of general movement patterns introduced and their subsequent refinement may, however, be closely related to the culture within which they live. This is a fascinating area and warrants further investigation. Notwithstanding the culture within which they live, physically literate individuals will be on a journey through which they are using an increasing range of movement patterns and capacities to effect. As adulthood and older age are reached competences are maintained, though they are possibly modified.

Challenges relating to dualism and elitism

In relation to the attribute focused on movement competence, issues have been raised about inferences of both dualism and elitism. However, physical literacy is neither a dualist nor an elitist concept. With respect to the first concern, it is misconceived to judge that specifically identifying physical competence in the concept is counter to monist principles. Monism does not prohibit attention being paid to the different dimensions that together comprise what it means to be human. The fundamental view of monism is that, at root, we are a single indivisible entity albeit comprising many different capabilities. These capabilities are interdependent and, essentially, function in close collaboration. The human being, viewed from a monist perspective, is a highly complex entity comprising capabilities which build from and mutually enrich each other. The concept of physical literacy identifies a specific capability that is intricately and significantly related to all other capabilities. It is accepted that in considering physical competence as a separate attribute, the functional aspects of the embodiment-as-instrument are highlighted. However, it is the case that we are manifest in a physical form and our physical competence is an important aspect of life.

With respect to elitism, as was set out in an early section of the book, physical literacy was developed partly to move on from the narrow association of embodied potential with elite performance. Physical literacy is in no way elitist; it can be achieved by all, and represents a capability fundamental to our human nature. The notion of physical competence in the definition needs to be understood in the context of individuals' endowment, particularly in respect of their unique embodied dimension. It is accepted that this makes assessment of physical literacy challenging in that it requires judgements of achievement to be made against individual progress and potential. This approach is contrary to much current practice in which achievement is matched against standards and norms. The notion of one directional progress 'up a ladder' is not the reality of developing movement competence, it more resembles the exploration of a three-dimensional climbing frame. In the context of physical literacy the notion of charting progress is more appropriate than assessment. An understanding of the range of movement vocabulary that can be developed, the various capacities that can be acquired and the ever more refined movement patterns that can be enacted, can create a scaffold within which the mover's physical literacy journey can be charted. Every individual is on a personal journey; the further each goes the richer the life opportunities. All individuals have movement potential and this should be carefully nurtured and celebrated as physical literacy is fostered.

Physically challenging situations

Thus far the chapter has looked at physical competence; however, the full definition of physical literacy goes beyond management of the embodied dimension per se and indicates that physically literate individuals can interact effectively, as appropriate to their endowment, with features in a wide variety of environments, and respond to situations that challenge their movement competence.

It is almost impossible to describe all the different types of environment with which individuals may need to interact and it is salutary to consider that each of these environments will 'call on' different and specific involvement of the embodied dimension. Table 5.1 is intended to reveal the wide variety of potential environments and to be an example of how these might be categorised. This is a complex exercise and the categories identified are neither mutually exclusive nor do they embrace every situation. Similarly the examples given are open to debate.

The progressive complexity of environments can be seen in Table 5.1. These range from situations where individuals move alone, without any equipment or apparatus in a predictable environment, through to highly unpredictable situations in which there may be interaction with others as well as the need to manage equipment and apparatus. In all cases the embodied dimension is intricately involved in effecting a productive relationship with the environment. The complexity of movement patterns and capacities that will need to be drawn on is vast. It is suggested that physically literate individuals will possess sufficient physical competence to achieve successful interaction in relation to challenges that are appropriate to their endowment. In addition, physically literate individuals will have the confidence borne of previous experience in the field of movement that has been effective and rewarding. They will not be daunted by new situations and challenges that are novel. The way this is realised is discussed in a later section of this chapter.

Physically literate individuals will be on a journey through which they are interacting effectively with features in an increasing range of environments. As adulthood and older age are reached the contexts for this interaction may alter, for example, through becoming more predictable.

Physical literacy and 'reading' the environment

Physically literate individuals endowed with a range of movement competences outlined at the start of this chapter should be able to achieve an effective and dynamic interaction within a wide variety of familiar and novel environments. The richer the vocabulary of competences, the better individuals will be able to respond to the embodied needs perceived in the environment. This is of significance, as was suggested earlier, on account of the fact that human beings develop and create themselves as a result of interactions with the environment. The ability to interact with the world is

Table 5.1 A categorisation of environments with examples from everyday life and physical activity settings

Nature of the environment	Examples from everyday life and situations other than structured physical activity settings	Examples from structured physical activity settings
An environment featuring gravitational force alone	Walking, running.	Forms of dance, martial arts and gymnastics
An environment featuring gravitational force plus different surfaces such as snow and ice, weather conditions, different media such as water	Walking on slippery ground or in a high wind, wading through water.	Skating, swimming, orienteering
An environment with fixed objects	Window cleaning, climbing a tree.	Some aspects of gymnastics, mountaineering, parkour, slalom skiing
An environment with heavy but moveable or semi-fixed objects	Furniture movingm using a see-saw, working a swing.	Weightlifting, bowls
An environment with portable objects to be carried, received or propelled	Carrying a tea tray or a suitcase, catching a falling plate.	Fielding in cricket, throwing/catching in netball, shot in athletics
An environment with instruments that require dexterous use	Operating a machine, playing a musical instrument, driving a car, writing with a pen.	Darts
An environment including an implement as an extension of the arm	Conducting an orchestra, chopping wood.	Using a ribbon in rhythmic gymnastics
An environment including using an implement as an extension of the arm in relation to a static object	Swatting a fly, cutting bread.	Golf, snooker
An environment including using an implement in relation to a moving object	Netting a butterfly.	Hockey, tennis, batting in cricket, clay pigeon shooting
An environment including others, with gravitational force alone	Negotiating a busy thoroughfare.	Group dance
An ever-changing environment including others, using an implement and/or portable object		Netball, basketball, hockey, lacrosse, fencing
A highly unpredictable environment often including others	Leaving a crowded building in the event of a fire.	Sailing, caving

referred to in the definition of physical literacy as 'reading' the environment. What is meant by the word 'read'?

It is useful here to consider what is meant by 'reading' in relation to the written word. Broadly, an ability to read could be described as indicating that an individual is able to give meaning to the written word and, furthermore, is able to relate separate items to each other, such as words, sentences and paragraphs, to make a coherent and meaningful whole. On these terms 'reading' goes beyond recognising individual words and requires an understanding or grasp of a passage or text. The reader is able to engage with the material that is read as it resonates with existing knowledge and experience. To do this the reader has to draw on a range of cognitive skills. New information connects with existing understanding and enriches the experience and knowledge base of the individual. Much of this takes place below the level of consciousness. In addition to being able to engage meaningfully with the written word the reader is able to respond verbally or in writing in order to articulate, develop or contest what has been read.

If this is translated into the context of physical literacy, the following picture emerges. The physically literate individual, on perceiving the environment, through a range of senses, appreciates, via experience, the relevant components of the display (e.g. shape size, weight, type of surface, speed, movement of others). These aspects of the environment are immediately grasped as meaningful, in that they resonate with embodied competences, and the individual will know intuitively how to move, to relate effectively with the combined aspects of the environment in question. The opportunities and challenges presented by the environment will be understood and will initiate an appropriate movement response. This ability to perceive the environment as 'matching' a particular motor response is the result of previous experience, and response is enacted to a considerable degree below the level of consciousness.

It is the case, however, that the mastery of much embodied 'reading' is acquired somewhat differently from early learning how to read the written word. Recognition of words is learned on a conscious level and only becomes pre-conscious or 'automatic' as the skill is mastered. In contrast, the foundation of embodied 'reading' is developed on a pre-conscious level as young children interact with the world around them. Through trial and error children build a vocabulary of movement patterns that correspond to, or are effective in relation to, features of the environment. Some of these patterns will be identified at a conscious level when language is understood and acquired. For example, parents and carers may draw attention to a child's ability to run, hop or skip or the need to move with care on a slippery surface, carry a delicate object gently, or use strength to lift a heavy book. However, more demanding and specialised embodied 'reading' will be acquired in the same way as learning to read the written word. That is, direct conscious instruction and practice will be needed as a complex movement pattern is learned. In this respect reading the written word and more sophisticated embodied 'reading' will function in a similar way; unfamiliar words and specific contextualised movement patterns will be acquired consciously, before becoming part of an individual's repertoire of intuitively used interactive abilities.

To understand the nature of embodied 'reading' of the environment it is useful to refer back to the discussion in Chapter 3 concerning embodied perception and response. As explained above 'reading' the environment incorporates both gathering information and acting on this information. The embodied relationship which individuals have with the world arises from the drive to interact with our surroundings defined as operative intentionality. As a result of operative intentionality objects are understood as having a particular meaning, that is 'operative meaning', being information about how individuals can relate to them physically.

As indicated in Chapter 3, this meaning is difficult to isolate as perception operates synaesthetically. In this process all sensory messages are immediately amalgamated. Individuals do not understand the nature of an object first through separate sensory modes and then have to piece together this information to create the object. An object is appreciated instantly as a whole. Information is gathered exteroceptively via senses such as sight and hearing as well as interoceptively. Interoceptive information about movement includes that from our sensory nerve endings that together give us a proprioceptive sense. Proprioception originates within our embodied dimension combining neural messages from nerve endings in the joints, the skin and the inner ear and provides an ongoing 'picture' of the position and movements of all parts of our embodied dimension. As individuals perceive an object or feature they 'read' the way they have interacted with it in the past. This information, or operative meaning, is elusive and often neglected on account both of a paucity of descriptive language and the way all sensory information is amalgamated.

It is of note that a range of contemporary philosophers have picked up the notions of operative intentionality and operative meaning and, in their different ways, given support for this perspective. Clark (1997) highlights the interplay between our embodied being and the world we inhabit in expressing the view that our behaviour patterns can be described as a 'dialogue' between ourselves and environmental factors. The idea is also put forward that in interacting with the world, it is not always our embodiment that leads the liaison; the world itself can initiate action. Clark (1997: 224) talks about a 'coupling' between an individual and his world, and explains that this coupling leaves much of our 'knowledge' out in the world. This knowledge, or operative meaning, is available for retrieval and is used as and when needed. Gibson (quoted in Weiss and Haber 1999: 129) takes this a step further and describes the information 'held' by the world as 'affordances'. He explains that 'Affordances may be defined . . . as opportunities for action in the environment of an organism'. He goes on to argue that objects in the environment are not inanimate features to which individuals ascribe an abstract concept, but are immediately meaningful. In a sense they 'engage' or 'communicate' with us, indicating how we can interact effectively with them.[1] Gill (2000) describes a symbiosis between our embodiment and the world, so intimate that there is not, and can never be, a clear distinction between the knower and the known.[2] Following from these insights there is a sense in which the world itself 'activates' particular aspects of our embodiment in order to establish an equilibrium between ourselves and the world. We 'know' immediately how to relate to an environment; appropriate embodied competences are 'alerted'; we feel 'at home' and able to interact with our surroundings.

As is indicated in the third attribute of physical literacy not only can physically literate individuals 'read' the physical environment, they are also able to respond appropriately with imagination and intelligence. This suggestion has some commonalities with notions discussed by other writers such as Best (1978: 58) and Arnold (1979: 17) who refer, respectively, to 'kinaesthetic intelligence' and 'intelligent action'. The imagination and intelligence alluded to in respect of physical literacy identifies the ability of the mover to select and enact an appropriate movement response to what is perceived. This will depend on the bank of movement responses that have already been developed and used and the ability to select and modify movement in the light of the specific needs of a situation. The bank of responses will in part reflect the range of environments within which the individual has interacted. The appropriateness of the response selected will depend on astute perception of the situation and the flexibility to bring into being newly refined movement patterns. These abilities are borne of experience and can demonstrate ingenuity and imagination. Confidence wrought from previous embodied interaction will enable the individual to interact effectively in ever more disparate and challenging situations. In achieving effective interaction in a novel environment, new meanings are created and a new blend of movement competences is added to the existing repertoire. As perceptual information expands and the bank of movement competences increases, the individual is ever more effective in interacting with situations that may be encountered.

Reading and responding to the environment in everyday situations and in physical activity settings

This aspect of physical literacy may be 'seen at work' in everyday situations and in physical activity settings. Reading the environment can be described from two perspectives. The first is perhaps easier to grasp because it can, to some extent, be described. In these situations it can be readily appreciated that individuals adapt their movement to the needs of the situation. Examples in everyday life will include care and caution in walking on an icy surface, carrying an unwieldy object and crossing a stream on stepping stones. In physical activity, examples are what is sometimes called 'reading the game' in a competitive context, and in outdoor events, such as sailing, responding appropriately to unpredictable environmental features such as wind and current. There is here, very often, a conscious realisation of the circumstances and some consideration and thought in moving in relation to them.

The second perspective in fact precedes the description above. Reading and responding to the environment in this sense refers to the way we as individuals interact fluently with our surroundings without having to stop and think. For example, we do not need to ask: 'How am I going to walk upstairs?', 'How am I going to dress myself?', 'How am I going to run for the bus?' In a physical activity context in which we are familiar we do not need to stop and think 'How am I going to catch the ball?', 'How am I going to do a forward roll?', 'How am I going to head the football' We carry out these habitual movements 'automatically', they are part of our repertoire of competences that are called on pre-reflectively as we encounter the challenges in the environment. In these situations individuals do not have to pay attention to their embodied interaction with the world. This is effected without conscious effort on account of the wealth of 'knowledge' held by our embodied dimension. Of course there are situations in which we may, indeed, ask such questions. If I had broken my leg I might well ask, 'How am I going to walk upstairs?' If there is a strong wind while I am playing tennis I would need to ask, 'How can I take account of the wind as I serve?', or if I was a newcomer to ball play I could indeed wonder, 'How am I going to catch the ball?' Characteristically this occurs in unfamiliar situations, in open skills and when individuals are in new physical activity settings. Once these new competences are grasped they tend to move 'down' to the pre-reflective level previously outlined.

Our ability to interact with the world is a fundamental aspect of being human and this ability lies at the heart of the value of physical literacy. The notion that a close relationship between our embodied dimension and the world which we inhabit is highly significant in our lives is succinctly expressed by Clark (1997: 98), who writes: 'Adaptive success finally accrues not to brains but to brain–body coalitions embedded in ecologically realistic environments.'

This section has proposed that physically literate individuals accrue an ever increasing bank of movement competences and a growing ability to interact with a wide range of environments. They will develop intelligent movement interaction with the world through perceptive reading of the environment and appropriate application of existing responses, effected alongside newly created responses where needed. These individuals will learn from all their interactions with the world, ceaselessly modifying and refining their response bank.

Recommended reading

Burkitt, I. (1999) *Bodies of Thought: Embodiment, Identity and Modernity*. Sage, London.

Clark, A. (1997) *Being There: Putting Brain, Body and World Together Again.* MIT Press, London, Chs 1, 2, 3, 5, 8 and Epilogue.

Gill, J.H. (2000) *The Tacit Mode.* State University of New York Press, New York, Chs 1, 2, 3, 5 and 6.

Whitehead, M.E. (2005a) Developing Physical Literacy. Paper given at Conference: PE for Today's Children. Primary Physical Education. Roehampton, July.

6 Physical literacy, the sense of self, relationships with others and the place of knowledge and understanding in the concept

Margaret Whitehead

Introduction

This chapter looks at the last three attributes of physical literacy. These are concerned with establishing a sense of self, developing fluent self-expression and effective communication with others, and acquiring knowledge in relation to movement and health.

The final three attributes of physical literacy (D, E and F) state that:

> *Physically literate individuals will have a well-established sense of self as embodied in the world. This, together with an articulate interaction with the environment, engenders positive self-esteem and self-confidence.*

> *Sensitivity to and awareness of our embodied competences leads to fluent self-expression through non-verbal communication and to perceptive and empathetic interaction with others.*

> *In addition, physically literate individuals will have the ability to identify and articulate the essential qualities that influence the effectiveness of their own movement performance, and have an understanding of the principles of embodied health with respect to basic aspects such as exercise, sleep and nutrition.*

The first three elements in the definition of physical literacy form the core of the capability. The final three attributes characteristically develop as motivation, confidence and physical competence and fluent interaction grow. As explained in Chapter 2, as individuals have rewarding experiences in respect of physical activity their sense of self and global self-confidence can be enhanced. In addition, awareness of the embodied dimension alongside a sound self-esteem can promote fluent self-expression and perceptive and empathetic interaction with others. Knowledge and understanding can be enriched by all aspects of participation.

In a reciprocal manner the final three attributes can have a positive effect on motivation, confidence, physical competence and fluent interaction with the environment. For example, an assured sense of self will feed into motivation and the willingness to accept challenges, while fluent interaction with others will add to confidence and the ability to work alongside others in physical activity settings. Similarly, knowledge and understanding will support the appreciation of developing physical competence and the perception of different environments.

Physical literacy and the development of a positive sense of self

It is suggested that in being physically literate, that is, being motivated to deploy one's physical competence and able to interact effectively with the environment, an individual's overall sense of self and self-esteem can be enhanced. This notion is in line with monist thinking and is not peculiar to the capability arising from our embodied dimension. From a monist perspective, which advocates the holistic nature of all human experience, the proposal that perceptions of our embodied dimension can feed into our sense of self would not be contested. In addition, referring back to the phenomenological and existentialist views that individuals create themselves from interaction with their surroundings, it follows that all aspects through which individuals interact with the world will play an ongoing part in the continual reaffirmation and re-creation of themselves. Our embodiment is undoubtedly a significant aspect of our personhood through which we interact with the world, and in this way this dimension of ourselves plays an important part in shaping our self-concept and our attitudes to ourselves. Physical literacy, incorporating the acquisition of embodied potential and the ready interaction with the world, provides a clear avenue through which individuals can develop a positive attitude towards themselves. This is developed further in Chapter 7.

It is interesting to note that early work in psychology in respect of a child's development of a sense of individual identity focused on the embodiment-as-object rather than on the embodied dimension as the source of a dynamic capability. The recognition of a 'mirror' image was championed as a critical moment at which time young children realised that they had a separate identity. There was no reference to any awareness of self before this 'seeing' in a mirror of the embodiment as a discrete object. It is therefore thought provoking to read some current views of philosophers and psychologists who move away from this position and advocate that self-awareness as an embodied being is evident long before the 'mirror image' stage (see also Whitehead 2005b). Gallagher (2005) has written extensively about the infant's body image and body schema and how these, in their different ways, make a significant contribution to the child's developing awareness of self. He also debates at length the experiences of using the embodied competences in providing both a sense of ownership and of agency. He argues that, from early infancy and before any development of a visual self through mirror images, children have what he calls a 'proprioceptive self'; that is, a sense of their own motor possibilities. Similarly, Burkitt (1999: 76) attributes the earliest form of self-awareness to the ability to move. He writes: 'The original sense of "I" is the "I can", a practical sense of the body's possibilities, and therefore the sense of identity possessed by humans is not based on disembodied thought, nor on early visual representation of the self.' For Burkitt individuals are first and foremost moving beings. Gallagher (2005: 9) goes further and suggests that our motile embodiment is the 'very thing that constitutes the self'. Indeed, he proposes that it is only via movement, via our embodiment, that individuals can begin to develop any sense of self.[1]

As this attribute of physical literacy indicates, the contribution to self-awareness and self-confidence does not lie only in the specific embodied self-awareness, but also in respect of the way that embodied competences enable individuals to develop effective relationships with the world. For those who are physically literate, self-confidence will grow as they readily interact with the world. There is a sense of self-affirmation in overcoming movement challenges, of whatever magnitude. These individuals are in tune with their surroundings. For the young or those with a particular disability, matching up to the demands of dressing themselves or for the adult the achievement of mastering the use of a new tool or scaling a difficult cliff face can each be hugely self-fulfilling and self-affirming. Burkitt (1999) takes this a step further in proposing that differing perceptions individuals have in respect of aspects of their embodiment may, on a conscious or pre-conscious level, influence their perceptual or emotional experience of the world.[2] The way in which attitudes to our embodied dimension affect our perception of the environment is an aspect of the concept that could well be developed.

The contribution to individuals' sense of self of a positive attitude to their dynamic embodied nature and a fluent interaction with the world does not diminish as they grow from early childhood through adulthood. For example, Burkitt (1999: 76) refers to how embodiment plays a key role in the ongoing development as individuals and writes, 'the sense of self we develop is primarily based on the feel we have of our body and the way it connects us to the world'. Gallagher re-enforces this view by putting forward the notion that via the ways in which the embodiment structures experience, our embodied presence in the world can shape human experience of self. These writers, with no axe to grind for participation in physical activity, put forward a clear case for attention to be paid to this mode of existence. Their work does not read as downplaying the physical dimension; rather their views suggest that human physicality should attract serious attention throughout the lifecourse.

There is also agreement that effective deployment of the embodied dimension can enhance self-esteem. Grogan (2008) outlines the positive effects exercise can have on mental health and well-being, and argues that exercise can be a way of improving self-esteem. This area is developed in Chapter 7. Grogan proposes that to have this beneficial effect, exercise should be more about enjoyment than about competition. Participants should have a positive experience with effective involvement and improvement being recognised, reinforced and rewarded. Gallagher (2005) refers specifically to the effects physical activity can have on self-perception and self-esteem. He writes:

> Exercise, dance, and other practices that affect motility and postural schemas can have an effect on the emotive evaluation of one's own body image. . ... Thus changes in the control of movement associated with exercise alter the way that subjects emotionally relate to and perceive their bodies.
>
> (Gallagher 2005: 144)

However, in the context of self-perception and self-esteem this positive attitude towards our embodied dimension has to incorporate an acceptance of our embodiment-as-object as well as an appreciation of the potentially fulfilling experiences that exercising this dimension of ourselves can bring. This, sadly, can present a problem in respect of developing physical literacy. It is the case that in Western culture there is an over-preoccupation with the embodiment-as-object. There are persistent messages sent out by the media presenting the ideal form that the female and the male embodiment-as-object should exhibit. This is an unrealistic paradigm for most and results in many people learning to see their embodied dimension as unsatisfactory and failing to match up to the ideals presented. Much has been written in texts on the sociology of the 'body' about the disturbing implications of this situation. What is even more worrying is the trend, in Western culture, towards individuals viewing themselves predominantly in terms of their embodiment-as-object. Low global self-esteem can be attributed in a great many cases to dissatisfaction with the embodiment-as-object and this is an unfortunate platform from which physical literacy has to build. Dismissal of their embodied dimension as less than ideal is not a good base from which to persuade people that the exercise of this dimension can be a rewarding and fulfilling experience. The public 'exposure' of their embodied dimension is a strong deterrent to participation in physical activity. Grogan (2008) urges that there should be a much more accepting attitude to variations in embodiment-as-object shapes and sizes, and also less focus on the aesthetics of the embodiment-as-object with more attention being paid to the functioning of this human dimension. The development of the concept of physical literacy is aimed, in part, at alerting people to the fact that there is far more to our embodiment than 'its' object form.

While recent writers in the field of sociology are often looking at embodiment-as-object satisfaction in relation to self-esteem, there is no doubt that they support participation in physical activity as of particular value in raising self-confidence. Experiences of those working with younger and older people would support this view. It is often seen that when individuals develop their embodied potential and master new competences there is a growth in self-confidence reflected beyond physical activity settings into other aspects of life. This may be in respect of meeting a movement challenge in everyday life or in a physical activity setting. There is some evidence that, in educational settings, the development of competence in structured physical activity can have a positive effect on self-confidence and on motivation in respect of learning generally. Performance and achievement in other areas of the curriculum can be enhanced, as can behaviour patterns and compliance in attending school. Examples of individuals who demonstrate this wider benefit may be found in Chapters 8, 10 and 11.

Given the views expressed in earlier chapters concerning the way in which our nature as embodied beings influences so much of our functioning as humans, these last findings come as no surprise. The development of any of our capabilities will have a far-reaching effect on our self-awareness, self-perception and self-confidence. Physical literacy is no exception. Indeed it could be argued that the way in which this capability has the potential not only to reaffirm the sense of self but also to enhance the relationship to the world, renders it of particular significance. The capability is fundamental to our functioning as human beings and is undoubtedly worthy of respect throughout the lifecourse.

However, it should be remembered that this heightened self-awareness and self-confidence is not restricted to physical literacy. It must surely be the case that in whatever sphere individuals operate, whichever of their capabilities they develop, there will be the potential for a positive impact on their total sense of self and self-esteem. A growing ability in respect of playing a musical instrument, grasping a foreign language or coming to terms with complex mathematical formulae would all seem to have the potential for a growth of self-respect. Physical literacy is not unique in having the possibility of enhancing quality of life; its uniqueness lies in the nature of the experiences that this capability offers. The focus of these experiences lies in active deployment of our embodiment, in capitalising on embodied potential.

Physical literacy, self-expression, self-presentation and interaction with others

This attribute of physical literacy builds from the aspect of the capability outlined above, in respect of developing a positive sense of self. This positive sense of self usually results in an assured self-presentation, realised both on account of global self-esteem, to which physical literacy can contribute and also because of the confidence individuals have of their embodied dimension. Individuals are not overly self-conscious in self-presentation and in no way display a self-deprecating attitude towards their embodied dimension. There is no divided attention between monitoring or judging themselves as seen by others and verbally presenting an idea or picking up information from the situation. There is a relaxed concentration on the task at hand with all aspects of their communication in harmony. Communication comprises verbal language, as well as gestures, posture and eye contact – to name only some of the elements of non-verbal communication. Nervous, self-conscious individuals with low self-esteem very often send out mixed messages in their verbal language and non-verbal behaviour. As Robertson (1989) explains the latter can become a message about the messenger rather than reinforcing whatever point is being made. For example, an apprehensive individual may be welcoming a visitor but instead of the embodied dimension displaying open, warm gestures, the movement behaviour may reveal cool and withdrawing characteristics. The effect can be easily felt by saying, 'How nice to see you' and at the same time folding one's arms and stepping backwards. The individual may well not be aware of the contradiction between the verbal and non-verbal communication being used. In other situations such as at an interview individuals may want to present a calm and confident persona but not be conscious that their gestures are agitated and their posture tight.

In contrast, physically literate individuals, in their self-expression and self-presentation, are likely to display a holistic quality, with verbal and non-verbal modes of communication re-enforcing each other. This facility may, in part, be the result of individuals having acquired a range of movement competences. This vocabulary will form a resource of movement possibilities from which an appropriate posture and mode of gesturing can be initiated. It is accepted that for those with a particular disability this expression of physical literacy will be less developed. However, self-confidence together with experience of a range of movement components, wherever an individual is on their physical literacy journey, can enhance assured self-presentation.

The second element in this attribute, concerned with perceptive and empathetic interaction with others, grows out of the confident and sensitive self-expression outlined above. Physically literate individuals can use the perceptive awareness of themselves to appreciate how others are feeling and thus respond appropriately. There is a sense in which physically literate individuals can 'identify with' the way others are presenting themselves and, as a result, can relate to others from a position of sympathetic understanding. There are a number of issues arising from this suggestion which will be considered briefly. These relate to scientific findings that explain how this sensitive interaction operates, to the way in which the embodied dimension lies at the heart of interpersonal relationships and to suggestions that this ability is evident in infants. Finally, the relationship of this facet of being physically literate to appreciation of the performing arts will be touched on.

Recent findings in neuroscience have begun to explain how fluent interaction can take place. Earlier chapters have explained the synaesthetic functioning of the senses in which all sensory information is understood 'as a whole' in creating whatever feature is being perceived. The separate senses are called 'modes' of perception and the merging of all the information perceived has been identified as 'intermodal' perception. An object or another person is consequently appreciated as a whole even if all aspects of what is perceived are not evident. This intermodal functioning also includes the interoceptive senses that inform individuals of the 'state' of their own embodied dimension. In a very complex way our bank of experiences, synaesthetically appreciated, provides a vehicle through which we can translate how others are looking and sounding into how they are feeling.[3]

This translation can be explained by what neuro-scientific theory has called 'mirror neurons'. These neurons link what is perceived of the other, to that which the perceiver has experienced, and enables the latter to 'put himself into the other's shoes'. The effect of mirror neurons is the creation of a situation in which viewing and perhaps hearing another person activates our own embodied systems, enabling us to 'mirror' the experience of others. Gallagher (2005: 50) explains that 'Neuronal patterns responsible for generating a motor image of an action are in large part the same neuronal patterns that are activated in the case of observing action and in performing action'. Mirror neurons activate an internal simulation of another person's behaviour through matching what is perceived with that which observers have experienced themselves. For example, Gallagher (2005: 102) explains: 'the same mirror neurons fire either when the subject *sees* a specific action such as grasping an object or the movement of hand to mouth performed by another person or when the subject *performs* the action herself'. It is argued that the brain areas that are responsible for planning an action are the same as those activated in the observation of others.

These insights are particularly pertinent to physical literacy in that they propose that effective social interaction is significantly affected by the embodied dimension. Indeed, Gallagher (2005) asserts that understanding the other person is primarily a form of intercorporeal interaction and presents a case in which individuals' embodied dimension provides primary access for understanding others. Two of his statements articulate this commitment. He writes (2005: 208) that 'The understanding of the other person is . . . a form of embodied practice', and again (2005: 27) that interpersonal interaction 'is a form of "body-reading" rather than mind reading'. In this way it is proposed that observers are not reading meaning directly from what is perceived of the other, but rather through an internal simulation of this to their own intermodal bank of experiences (see also Whitehead 2005b). The observer is not interacting directly with the other person so much as interacting with 'an internally simulated model of himself' (Gallagher 2005: 222). It is not difficult, therefore, to conceive of the situation in which the richer the intermodal bank of experiences the richer will be the vocabulary of potential 'matches' with what is perceived in others. Gallagher goes on to suggest that this intermodal interaction is a fundamental capacity with which individuals are endowed at birth. Referring to recent research, he writes:

> At 5–7 months infants are able to detect correspondences between visual and auditory information that specify the expression of emotions.

Importantly, the perception of emotion in the movement of others is a perception of an embodied comportment, rather than a theory or simulation of an emotional state.

(Gallagher 2005: 227)

There is a sense in which, even at this stage, infants use awareness of their embodied self to 'understand' the embodied actions of others. Infants do not play a passive role when they observe others; they are in a dynamic interaction with them. As young children observe, they experience different aspects of being and thus begin to build up their repertoire of perceptions. Gallagher explains that the way the embodiment is used in early interaction with others provides the primary access individuals have for understanding other people, and this use of the embodied dimension persists throughout life.

Looking beyond these early years it would seem to be the case that what we understand of others depends on what we have come to appreciate in ourselves. Indeed, it would seem that the more individuals come to know themselves as embodied, the better they are able to read off nuances of the experiences of others. It is pertinent that Gallagher also claims that effective interaction with others depends to a significant degree on the acuteness of the observer's perception of their own embodied dimension. It is not surprising therefore that he suggests that those who find it difficult to develop inter-personal relationships may have problems with their own motor abilities, may lack rich intermodal experience and/or have less effective mirror neurons. Referring to these neurons in respect of autism he suggests that:

Just these kinds of sensory-motor processes have been shown to be important in explaining some basic aspects of social cognition. Here the evidence that a subject's understanding of another person's actions and intentions depends to some extent on a mirrored reverberation in the subject's own motor system is relevant.

(Gallagher 2005: 232)[4]

In addition to this matching of experiences, it is proposed that in interacting with others we both refer back to our bank of existing experiences and add to that bank of data. Not only does the acuteness of our sensitivity to and management of our embodiment affect sensitivity to and empathy with others, perception of others can, in a reciprocal way, enrich the perception we have of ourselves.

It is thought provoking that the theories set out above would seem to explain individuals' response to watching the performing arts. There has been a long-held view that there is some kind of proprioceptive appreciation of, or empathy with, the movement of a performing artist in, for example, dance and drama, and furthermore that those with richer movement experiences can have a 'better' appreciation of the artistic enterprise. This has formerly been discounted as there were seen to be no grounds on which this claim could be verified. With the research on mirror neurones there is support for the validity of this notion. It is perhaps not too bold to suggest that a physically literate individual with a substantial bank of movement components can have a richer experience of watching the performing arts. In addition, there is the reciprocal effect that occurs in interaction as mentioned above. In the context of watching performing art presentations not only can individuals empathise with what the performer is expressing, but observers' sensitive perception and appreciation can actually add to their own repertoire of feelings and emotion. Thus physically literate individuals can have a richer experience of an art form and come away from the encounter having added to their own wealth of sensibilities.

This chapter so far has argued that physically literate individuals equipped with a sound sense of self can express themselves fluently and can draw on their embodied experiences and perceptions to foster understanding and empathetic relationships with others. This last, it was argued, is evident even in very young children and is the foundation of interaction with others throughout life.

Physical literacy and propositional knowledge

The issue of the role of propositional knowledge, involving language and understanding, in respect of being physically literate, presents a challenge to the concept. As was outlined in Chapter 2, discussion of the concept requires a change in the way we normally talk and think about our embodied dimension. Physical literacy is a capability the understanding of which demands an appreciation that spans both the pre-reflective and the reflective aspects of human embodied functioning; that is, both the embodiment-as-lived and the concrete embodied form. A new discourse is needed to move on from language forms commonly used in Western culture that seem only to have one way to refer to our embodied dimension, that is, as an object. The notion of our having an 'embodied dimension' that functions on two 'levels' is not part of everyday language, the term used to refer to this aspect of our human condition, being the 'body'. The 'body' is classified as a noun, a thing, an 'it', and it will be a huge task to change both the appreciation of our embodied dimension and the habitual way to which 'it' is referred. It is clearly one of the challenges of the concept of physical literacy to 're-educate' people to realise that there is more to their embodiment than just an object to be dressed, fed and medically cared for.

In this context therefore, to suggest that physical literacy itself should include an attribute which is very likely to use dualist language is clearly problematic. It is fascinating to learn from Brownell (1995) that the Chinese have three words for the 'body', each recognising a different mode of embodiment. These are 'shen' – the animate embodiment-as-lived; 'ti' – the inanimate embodiment-as-object or instrument; and 'shi' – the embodiment-as-corpse. Sadly in the English language we do not have the options of 'ti' and 'shen', habitually referring to our embodied dimension as 'ti'. The view of our embodiment taken in respect of physical literacy draws on both 'ti' and 'shen', arguing that, while they are different modes of the embodiment, they are inextricably interconnected in relation to our functioning as human beings.[5] There is an intriguing story told by Csordas (in Weiss and Haber 1999: 143) which refers to a discussion between a Western anthropologist and a philosopher from New Caledonia, in which the latter indicated that before their primitive tribe had contact with the West, his people had not formed a concept of the embodiment-as-object, as they were living their lives in a totally holistic mode. In fact they did not have a word for their embodiment as a separate entity. On enquiring what Western thought had brought to his people the philosopher replied, 'What you've brought us is the body.'[6]

There is something of an irony in any doubt about the place of movement knowledge, understanding and language in respect of being physically literate. As was indicated in Chapter 4, very many of the concepts which individuals use in everyday language are grounded in our embodied interaction with the world. It is suggested (Lakoff and Johnson 1999) that concepts such as up, down, above, below, near and far are not grasped until the corresponding interaction with the world via our embodied dimension has been experienced. And again, far from aspects of movement appreciation being foreign to our language, our speech is imbued with movement metaphors. Individuals talk of being *weighed down* with responsibilities, having *close* friends, feeling *down* when they are depressed and describing a colleague's understanding of a subject as *way ahead* of their own. All the words in italics are metaphors based on movement experiences.

In developing the concept of physical literacy it has never been a goal to downplay the importance of our embodiment-as-instrument, or in other words our physical presence in the world, but rather to add a further facet to the perception of the embodied dimension. In very many situations it is both appropriate and important to view the embodiment objectively. For example, this is the view individuals take when learning a new movement pattern, and the perspective which individuals expect a doctor, dentist or physiotherapist to take on their embodiment.

The attribute of physical literacy concerned with the acquisition of knowledge and understanding has two constituents. The first is concerned with grasping the essential principles of movement and performance. It would seem uncontroversial to expect physically literate individuals to have an appreciation of the basic components of movement, and to be able to evaluate their own performance and that of others. This will involve the use of appropriate vocabulary as well as some ability to observe movement. Where possible this ability should extend first into a simple diagnosis of what is making a movement more or less effective and then into an understanding of how to improve and develop the movement pattern or skill. Requirements specified for school-based curriculum physical activity in England (QCA 2007) endorse this aspect of physical literacy and include among their aims the development of 'the knowledge and understanding of what needs to be achieved and . . . ways to promote improvement'. In the context of physical literacy as a self-motivated lifelong involvement in physical activity it is clearly important for individuals to be able to take some responsibility for their own movement. Much activity throughout life will not be monitored by a teacher or coach, and individuals will need to evaluate their own performance and take steps to effect an improvement.

The second aspect of knowledge and understanding is concerned with health and fitness, and sees the physically literate individual as having a basic understanding of issues such as the value of exercise, appropriate diet and the need for relaxation and sleep. Curriculum requirements in England (QCA 2007) again endorse this view, and include the statement that pupils should 'Understand that physical activity contributes to the healthy functioning of the body and mind and is an essential component of a healthy lifestyle'. This knowledge and understanding will start from a very simple base in the early years with young children appreciating the effect that exercise has on aspects of their embodiment such as the heart and the lungs, and will gradually become more sophisticated, where this is feasible, in appreciating more complex aspects of health and fitness.

Indeed, in taking responsibility for their health and well-being it is essential that individuals adopt an 'objective' view of themselves in deciding how best to manage aspects of life. It would be unacceptable for the concept of physical literacy to omit the care, attention and respect individuals should show to their embodied dimension as an instrument or mechanism. There is much debate in Western culture about, for example, the amount of exercise individuals should take, the nature of the food they should eat and the types of medication they should use. It therefore has to be accepted that to be physically literate in our culture, with its sophisticated knowledge of all aspects of health, one would require a basic understanding of the principles of embodied health with respect to areas such as exercise, sleep and nutrition. That having been said it has to be remembered that in including this attribute of physical literacy there will be a tension between the discourse used generally in respect of the concept and that used in everyday language.

Notwithstanding the expectations discussed above, the attribute of physical literacy concerned with knowledge and understanding does not demand the grasp of technical biomechanical and medical scientific concepts, but sufficient understanding to appreciate both how movement is structured and the importance of care of the embodiment-as-instrument. Two other areas of debate have arisen in respect of this attribute. The first concerns whether, to be physically literate, individuals need to have an appreciation of their nature as beings-in-the-world and the role played in existence by the embodiment at a pre-reflective level. The answer to this question must be in the negative, as these notions are complex and somewhat abstract. Some broad appreciation could be an asset but it would not seem essential to have grasped existential and phenomenological principles to be physically literate. However, a sound understanding of the underlying philosophical principles on which physical literacy is based would seem to be desirable, if not essential, for practitioners working to promote physical literacy in physical activity settings. The second area of debate is whether individuals can be physically literate if they have achieved this attribute but none of the others. In other words: 'Can physical literacy be a purely intellectual achievement?' The answer is again in the negative, as at the heart of physical literacy are the motivation, confidence and physical competence that promote an active and lifelong involvement in some form or forms of structured physical activity.

The description of physically literate individuals that has been developed through the course of Part I of this volume reveals that each is on a personal journey, as appropriate to their endowment. Each will grow in motivation, in confidence and physical competence and in the ability to interact with a wider variety of environments. Each will realise enhanced self-esteem and will grow in confident self-presentation and empathetic interactions with others. Each will gradually accrue wider and deeper knowledge and understanding of the nature of movement and of the relationship between physical activity and health and well-being. Each physically literate individual will experience an enhanced quality of life, having capitalised on one of their innate human dimensions.

Recommended reading

Burkitt, I. (1999) *Bodies of Thought: Embodiment, Identity and Modernity*, Sage, London, Ch. 4.

Gallagher, S. (2005) *How the Body Shapes the Mind*, Clarendon Press, Oxford, Chs 6 and 9.

Whitehead, M.E. (2007d) Physical literacy: philosophical considerations in relation to developing a sense of self, universality and propositional knowledge. *Sport, Ethics and Philosophy*, 1, 3: 281–298.

Part II

Contextual connections

7 The physical self and physical literacy

Kenneth Fox

Introduction

The aim of this chapter is to provide an outline of key concepts underpinning the nature of the physical self in terms of its content, structure and its relationship with self-esteem. The intention is to offer a framework that will stimulate and facilitate discussion about how physical literacy might interweave with self-perceptions. Importantly, it provides the theoretical background to the discussion of physical literacy and the development of a positive sense of self in Chapter 6. This chapter assimilates theoretical concepts with empirical research conducted over the past twenty years on physical self-perceptions, described in greater detail in Fox and Wilson (2008). It is written primarily from the perspectives of social psychologist, human developmentalist, teacher/educator and parent.

Conceptual and definitional issues around the self

The first challenge facing the student of self is presented by the large volumes of diverse literature. It has been a central topic in disciplines as diverse as philosophy, sociology, psychology, theology and even economics. This is hardly surprising given that as society has passed through and beyond modernity, the individual has increased in prominence as a unit of analysis in social theory. Granted at least the impression of greater individual autonomy in society, reflected in contemporary political intentions and strategies to offer *choice,* the self has become central to understanding decision-making and motivation. Clear evidence exists to show that self-perceptions influence both choice of and persistence in a diverse range of behaviours from supermarket purchases, career pathways to friendships. Whether or not we apply effort to participate in physical activity or sport, try hard in school or at work, or go out of our way to be accepted by a particular friendship group is strongly related to both personal aspirations and self-perceptions of ability.

Furthermore, what we feel about ourselves has increasingly been seen as an important contributor to both our capacity to achieve and our mental health status. High self-esteem is often seen as a component of psychological well-being and is accompanied by emotional stability and thus a stronger base from which to grow and learn. Low self-esteem is a symptom of common mental disorders such as depression, instability and unhappiness. As a result, self-perceptions and self-esteem are directly or indirectly targeted in many therapeutic and educational programmes.

Language and labelling divergences in the self literature have handicapped our capacity to find common understanding and solutions to the nature of the self and the mechanisms through which it operates. However, in recent years, several definitions and themes have emerged that are becoming more broadly accepted within and across disciplines. Self-concept may be seen frequently used, particularly in the literature prior to the 1990s. It is an all-encompassing term that summarises how the individual self-describes. This might combine personality traits such as 'I am honest, friendly, or not very reliable'; roles in life (sometimes termed identities) such as 'I am a father, son, student'; competencies such as 'I am strong, clever, shy'; or features such as 'I am tall, young and skinny'. Self-esteem in contrast is an evaluative statement about worth as a person. It therefore carries emotional implications so that high self-esteem is accompanied by a sense of personal pride and optimism whereas low self-esteem can bring about feelings of shame and hopelessness. The healthy human drive is therefore to seek out opportunities to experience good feelings about the self. Where this goes wrong, and, given the burgeoning mental illness prevalence, this seems to be common, we see symptoms of depression such as unhappiness, anxiety, apathy, withdrawal, over-defensiveness, worthlessness and self-loathing. In extreme cases this may contribute to substance abuse and self-harm.

Self-direction and enhancement

There has been a strong belief among many social psychologists since the early writings of James (1892) that the self has two elements. The self-director or the 'I' provides an ongoing dynamic subjective summary of the activities, competencies and achievements of the objective self known as the 'Me'. The self-director is the cognitive core of the self or the control console that attempts to synthesise the components of the self and its life interactions. It summarises its achievements and makes overall statements about its worth, one of which is self-esteem. The best measures of self-esteem used by psychologists avoid reference to specific life domains such as friendships, work or physical characteristics and feature items about self-respect, worth and general feelings of success, and thus tap into what is known as global self-esteem.

This approach is critical because individuals and different population subgroups vary in the sources and weighting of information about themselves used to judge their worth. Younger generations may be more concerned about their physical appearance such as keeping slim or presenting their hair in a fashionable way. For older populations, friendships or making a positive contribution to local communities may be more important. Competencies and attributes that are highly valued at the societal or subgroup level will influence which criteria are used by individuals to judge their self-worth. The degree to which the individual bows to those societal demands is an assessment of conformity with those who are excessively submissive possibly labelled as 'slaves to fashion' or 'having no mind of their own'. Those rejecting societal values are at best categorised as 'individualistic' and at worst 'weird' or 'eccentric'.

In line with the positive human drive to feel good about self, the self-director when working effectively can operate self-serving strategies that maximise positive outcomes and minimise negative impacts (see Fox 1997 for greater detail). One such technique involves selection and biasing of information so that the self takes more responsibility for success than failure. Another is to direct efforts into behaviours that yield success and to avoid those that produce a sense of failure. Where there is no choice but to be involved, it is possible to discount the importance of engagement or denigrate the activity and not make an effort, thus avoiding any exposure of inadequacy. This is a common feature in schools where low competence in a school subject might be discounted by attaching little value in importance. When youngsters indicate that they are not interested in a school subject, they may be expressing the view that they have been forced to discount its importance because they do not feel that they are competent.

Ultimately, through its managerial role, the self-director has two major tasks. It has to develop a sense of coherence of self and a core identity that is stable across settings. This is important for the projection of an identity and to establish personality or individuality, and to provide a consistent and predictable canvass with which others can interact. This allows healthy human relationships to blossom and mature. Once a sound and harmonious core is established, the individual is better equipped to take on challenges, to explore, to stretch boundaries, to learn from difficult situations and to continue to grow. These tasks feature heavily in adolescence where youngsters are trying to find out who they are and what they want to be seen as. In experimentation, risk-taking and butterfly-like behaviour where life sampling is occurring, setbacks and mood swings are commonplace. Parents and teachers who understand these behaviours, who avoid overreacting and who apply a degree of sensitivity tend to be more helpful than those who attempt to be more controlling (see Fox 2009 for a more detailed discussion on parenting for physical activity).

The development of the self-system

The self is therefore best seen as a dynamic system which is constantly reacting and adjusting to life experiences, particularly in youth. This notion has been supported by many theorists including Harter (1996), Epstein

(1991), Markus and Wurf (1987) through their self-schemata theory, and Deci and Ryan (1995, 2002) through self-determination theory that will be addressed in greater detail later.

Before the 1980s, the concept of multidimensionality of self emerged. In contrast to seeing the self as a unified whole, psychologists such as Shavelson, Hubner and Stanton (1976) began to describe multifaceted hierarchical models of the self. A generalised self-concept or self-esteem was at the apex and this was underpinned by perceptions in different life domains such as school work or occupation, spirituality, friendships and the physical self. Beneath these domains were perceptions in more specific sub-domains such as mathematics or English ability, same- or opposite-sex friendships, physical appearance and physical ability. The notion was that experiences in these specific domains may generalise, if repeated often enough, to higher, more general levels of self. Perhaps then, educational programmes could help children experience positive self-perceptions in these domains and subsequently facilitate the development of a strong sense of self and higher self-esteem.

However, it takes time for the complexity of the self-system to develop. Young children (aged 5 to 8 years) generally have very simple perceptions of themselves. They have limited experience and probably capacity to judge their levels of ability or their characteristics in relation to others. They focus on the 'here and now' and what can be seen. They have little capacity to perceive abstractions such as health and largely operate on a 'good boy-bad boy' level of reasoning whereby their behaviour is regulated externally to please or comply with others. Measurable at this age are perceptions of appearance, characteristics such as height or abilities such as running speed, and to a lesser extent abilities in school work and popularity in friendships. Of course physical appearance and sports activity are very public and so are particularly salient. However, perceptions at this age are not sophisticated and are frequently inaccurate on the side of being overly optimistic. Young children do not have a strong grasp of the concept of ability differences among their peers and believe that the best performers are successful because they are trying hard. They are therefore highly motivated, apply effort and are keen to please those around them such as parents and teachers. To some extent, it is a shame that this positive but naïve psychological state does not last.

As children develop (ages 9 to 12 years), they learn to compare their abilities and become more accurate in their estimates. They also become more capable of differentiating their performances in a wider range of domains such as school work, friendships, appearance and physical abilities (Nicholls 1989). It becomes possible to tap into a generalised or global self-esteem which can reflect their emotional states. They start to realise that a combination of effort and ability produces successful performance and this starts to seriously influence their level of motivation. If they perceive low ability in, for example, playground football, and that their efforts cannot overcome this, then they become at risk of developing learned helplessness. This is a state where the belief dominates that 'no matter how much I try, it does not make a difference, so why should I bother trying any longer?' It is easier to drop out. Sadly this is all too evident in respect of participation in physical activity both in later childhood, youth and adulthood.

Adolescence sees the development of a more complex adult-like self-system that can be made up of perceptions in many different life domains. Harter's Self-Perception Profile for Adolescents (1988) attempts to assess perceptions of competence in twelve life arenas. Adolescence is a time when the self-director is hard at work. Havighurst (1972) has suggested that the key tasks of adolescence are to find and establish identity. Young people of this age have a sense of self-esteem but can be inconsistent and moody as they seek to find where they belong.

Self-perceptions remain predictive of behaviours throughout life. In older age, for example, there is a strong drive to feel that growth and learning is still taking place (Stathi *et al.* 2002). The need for a sense of personal achievement does not necessarily decline and remains part of subjective well-being. Indeed, the loss of opportunity to successfully and independently manage daily life through physical or mental incapacity may be an important contributor to the higher levels of depression in older adults. Remaining active and socially involved is a key to mental health in older people. It helps prevent and delay the onset of dementia and to maintain physical function. The concept of physical literacy therefore is equally relevant for older as for young people. This area is discussed more fully in Chapter 10.

The physical self

With the recognition of multidimensionality of the self-system came greater attention to its parts. Physical aspects of the self featured consistently as an important element. This is not surprising given that the physical self is visible and provides the primary means of face-to-face interactions. The physical self has been likened to the 'public self', since it is provides a vehicle for important human functions such as sustenance, expression, sexuality and celebration.

Building on early work by Sonstroem (1978), Fox and Corbin (1989) more systematically analysed the structure and content of the physical self. Using open-ended interviews and questionnaires, they asked young men and women what made them feel good and bad about their physical selves and how this might influence how they felt about themselves overall. The outcome was the development of the Physical Self-Perception Profile (PSPP) (Fox 1990), which provides a means of assessing perceived competence or adequacy in the sub-domains of physical strength, physical condition, appearance of the body and sports competence. A physical self-worth subscale is included to represent an overall judgement of the physical self similar to a domain-specific version of global self-esteem. Along similar lines the Physical Self-Description Questionnaire was developed by Marsh *et al.* (1994). These instruments have been used widely in research and have been translated into many different languages. Different versions have been developed for children and other groups in order to better understand how the physical self works and how it varies from population to population. Several key findings have emerged from over a hundred studies using these instruments.

1.   The physical self is closely related to global self-esteem with correlations in the region of r = 0.6–0.7. It is also related to other indicators of psychological health such as emotional stability. Programmes that target physical self-perceptions may be used to improve self-esteem and mental health.
2.   Physical self-perceptions closely predict amount and type of involvement in physical activity and sport. There is some evidence of a causal effect in young people, suggesting that programmes need to consider their effect on physical self-perceptions in order to engage participants in physical activity.

These two findings would seem to underwrite the importance of developing and maintaining those attributes of physical literacy that are concerned with motivation, confidence and self-esteem. Key here is the nature of the relationship between the participant and the practitioner overseeing the activity. This point is picked up later in this chapter and in Chapter 14.

The role of perceived importance

The concepts of value and importance touched upon earlier in this chapter have also been applied in the physical domain. In James' early work (1892), self-esteem was seen to be the outcome of a ratio between competencies and ambitions or aspirations. In short, he believed that our level of self-esteem is dependent on the degree to which we feel we are able to be the person we want to be. In aspects of life where individuals perceived a need to aspire but feel inadequate, then low self-esteem would be experienced and high self-esteem would result from competence leading to achievement and the meeting of goals and aspirations.

This hypothesis has been operationalised by social psychologists as the assessment of perceived importance to self of aspects of life. Following Harter's lead, Fox and Corbin developed a Perceived Importance Profile (PIP) alongside the PSPP to measure the importance to self of each of the four PSPP sub-domains. Where high importance was attached to a low competence domain, then a discrepancy resulted, reflecting that aspirations were not being met. Consistently across several studies, in different countries and languages, those with higher discrepancy scores have lower physical self-worth and lower global self-esteem.

There is good evidence of discounting the importance of physical activity and sport competence in adolescent girls and a sector of boys. If low importance can be attached to a particular perceptual domain such as physical competence, then low competence will not matter. Where participation remains compulsory such as in physical education, it is not surprising that an expression of low importance is seen by a regular supply of excuse notes, applying minimal effort in activities, or simply declaring 'I ain't bovvered'.

Herein exists a dilemma for the educator or health promotion specialist. Discounting areas of low competence may provide at least some temporary protection for the self and mental well-being. If we can feel good about all our competencies and forget about our weaknesses, then life should be better. However, for other aspects of health and well-being, we need to encourage youngsters to remain engaged with their physical skills for as long as is possible. Certainly the tenets of physical literacy would suggest that this is essential. This would suggest that strategies are required to help youngsters avoid discounting of skills in areas where there are broader benefits to their selves and health. This is particularly the case where youngsters are still growing and developing as future ability is not predicted well by current ability. Physical competence and fitness have the potential to make a very important contribution.

Furthermore, there are areas of self, particularly in the physical domain, which are difficult to discount. In adolescent and young adult females, the primary source of discrepancy comes from a mismatch between perceived physical attractiveness and the importance of attractiveness or 'looking good'. Boys also suffer but to a lesser degree.

In this case, societal values, reflected in icons, language and status, emphasise that the body needs to look slim, toned and attractive. If youngsters feels unhappy with their bodies, and research has shown that this is the case for the large majority of adolescent girls (Hill 2006), then the opportunity to discount the importance of looking good is unlikely to be available to them. Society is too dominant to allow this to influence all but the very strong-willed or individualistic youngster, who perhaps has a robust enough sense of self in other areas of life or a personality type to equip them to deal with this discrepancy.

It appears then that levels of perceived competence or adequacy do not provide the full explanation of self-esteem. Perceived importance, which is a kind of value, may also provide an influence. Although this notion is intuitively plausible, it remains controversial as not all statistical approaches to date have yielded full support (Marsh and Sonstroem 1995). However, it is clear that for a complete understanding of self-perceptions and their influence on behaviours and mental well-being, how individuals are influenced by, and deal with, societal values and dictates in relation to their own values is critical. This is likely to be particularly important for young people, as they are still in the process of formulating their own value systems.

The physical self and engagement in physical activity

The physical self may be seen as a central mediator in choice and persistence in physical and social activities. Following the self-enhancement strategies operated by the self-director, there will be a strong tendency to drive the self to engage in activities which yield a sense of high perceived competence and success. This falls in line with competence motivation theory (Harter 1978) and applies to the full range of physical endeavours such as dance or musical performance, competitive sports, fitness activities, running, cycling or swimming. It will also explain engagement in activities such as weight lifting, modelling and cheerleading that allow valued attributes of the physical self to be displayed or expressed. Conversely, areas of life which bring a sense of inadequacy, stress or embarrassment will tend to be avoided so that those who are not proud or who are ashamed of their physical selves will avoid settings such as dance or swimming that require public display.

Research has consistently revealed that people who report higher levels of perceived physical competence are much more likely to be physically active. The causal direction of this relationship is unclear but there is likely to be a two-way iterative process in operation. On the one hand, there is a natural attraction to and engagement in activities where competence can be expressed so that the drive of energy originates from self-perceptions. Ironically, sports clubs and fitness gyms will attract those who already feel good about their abilities. This motivational force has often been termed 'self-enhancement' and is largely driven from within the individual. On the other hand, engagement in practice, being coached and playing regularly is likely to build skill and also self-perceptions of competence. The motivational force in this case has been termed 'skill enhancement'. This process is very much behind teaching and health programmes that are designed to build physical skill, decision-making and self-confidence.

Whichever directional drive is in operation, by the time youngsters leave school, it is possible to predict 70 to 80 per cent of their degree of engagement in sport and exercise simply from their score on a physical self-perception profile. This effect can remain throughout life with middle-aged adults reporting that they are not active for health 'because I am not the sporty type' (The Sports Council and Health Education Authority 1992). In older people, confidence in the ability to walk unassisted and unaccompanied and independently to complete the daily tasks of living becomes important.

Growing up is therefore a critical time for building physical self-perceptions, and this in turn can influence engagement in physical activity and sport throughout life. The youngster who drops out early will not benefit from further support and is unlikely to improve in comparison to those selected for teams. In an unmanaged system, therefore, it is easy to see that an upward or downward spiral can develop whereby the skill-rich become richer and the skill-poor become poorer. This can have a lasting effect. Once a non-sporty or active identity forms in a person, it will take a powerful intervention to change this perception. Conversely, once a positive exercise or sport identity is formed, then it tends to feed itself. Individuals who view themselves as an athlete or a dancer will tend to invest in the subculture by choosing similar friends, buying clothes that fit the image and behaving in ways that the subculture expects.

Enhancing and developing the physical self

There is scope for parents, partners, leaders, teachers and peers to help people, throughout the lifecourse, to realise a positive physical self and self-esteem. This area is developed in Chapters 13 and 14 (see also Whitehead with Murdoch 2006). Throughout the social psychology literature several key elements of human emotional need emerge, regardless of age group, that are important for well-being. These are:

- the need to feel competent
- the need to feel autonomous
- the need to feel a sense of significance
- the need to feel a sense of belonging.

The physical self may play an important role in the development of some of these needs. The development of physical abilities seems an obvious route through which to help people feel competent and experience psychological well-being. However, this is not quite as simple as it sounds. Competence is often judged by the individual or society through comparison with others of similar age and gender. As reported earlier, intuitive judgement of performances through comparison with those around them starts in children in the later years of primary school. For example, children become gradually more accurate at ranking themselves among their classmates. They soon come to realise who are the most athletic and physically competent, who has less or more attractive features, who are the most popular children and who is the most clever. Clearly, those who are publicly ranked high are more likely to develop the strongest sense of perceived competence. These youngsters will also be first to be selected for teams and be publicly acclaimed when they do well. Excellence by its definition suggests exclusivity, as it is based on unusual, remarkable and outstanding performance. Perceived competence based solely on comparisons of this nature suggests that it is accessible only to those who are more gifted.

Fortunately, in applying achievement goal theory in the physical activity context, researchers such as Duda *et al.* (1992) and Roberts (1992) have identified that it is possible to concurrently hold two schema or lay theories that allow a sense of competence in this activity to be developed. The first which is based on external referencing through peer or norm comparisons has been termed ego orientation. Using this perspective, in order to feel competent, it is necessary to at least believe that your performance is superior to those around you. The alternative is mastery or task orientation, where the individual focuses more directly on self-comparison and personal improvement. Success is judged as the mastery of tasks such as learning a physical activity or being able to walk uphill that little bit further than before in attempts to become fitter. The beauty of a mastery orientation is that it is accessible to all, regardless of initial ability levels. It marries well with the notion that individuals are on their own physical literacy journey and that physical literacy is concerned with personal participation and mastery rather than achieving in comparison with others.

However, the world is competitive by nature and selection operates overtly through comparisons among individuals, whether it be in physical competence, fitness, sport, looking for a partner or for a job. It is therefore not surprising that ego perspectives can dominate. The effective teacher, parent or leader counterbalances this by constantly emphasising the importance of focusing on personal improvement and mastering skills and tasks. Comparison with others is discouraged because effort applied to personal progress is the key to long-term motivation and change. Even top-level sportsmen and women apply this approach as it drives them through the tedium of practice and training and also helps provide a buffer when they are beaten in competition. A mastery approach is therefore critical in helping people experience competence. It has been found that this is important throughout the lifecourse and in different cultures. In order to experience subjective well-being, for example, older adults need to feel that they are learning, developing and growing in terms of their abilities (Stathi *et al.* 2002; Po-Wen Ku *et al.* 2007).

In a world where we are seduced through media images (and which are often artificially modified) to aspire to unrealistically high standards of appearance, then perhaps the same self-referenced approach is needed. Too many young people grow through adolescence disliking the shape, size and appearance of their 'bodies' (Hill 2006) to the point, where the 'body' becomes an unwelcome element of the self. Unless ways can be found of helping young people accept themselves as they are and celebrate their uniqueness and individuality, then many will progress through life with feelings of low self-confidence and introspection. Of course, this raises important issues about approaches to helping people who are overweight or obese deal with a condition that is potentially damaging to health. A dilemma arises for health professionals. Raising awareness of the condition can increase feelings of insecurity and guilt. Yet something needs to be done if action is to be taken to put the situation right. Adopting a mastery approach would focus attention on encouraging effort and securing the behaviours that can rectify the condition such as physical activity and healthy eating. A short- and long-term goal-setting approach for personal mastery would be applied. Examples of this approach are discussed in Chapter 8. Of course the concept of embodiment featured in the physical literacy approach perfectly fits with such a notion. Where the body is experienced as integral to the self rather than as a physical appendage to the self, then a more wholesome, rounded interface with life might be achievable.

Not only is it important to feel competent, but critical to self-esteem is the feeling of ownership of success. Put succinctly, 'it's not just that I *did* it, it's that I did it'. This is termed by psychologists as an aspect of self-determination or autonomy. People need to feel that they are empowered and in charge of their destiny. In order to encourage a sense of autonomy, teachers, helpers and parents need to look at how their interactions can hand over a sense of ownership for success. Traditionally the professional role of doctor, nurse, coach, and to some extent teacher has been counterproductive here. Professionals can often set themselves up as the white-coated experts who are the source of all knowledge. They cure, prescribe, train, coach or teach in a way that encourages the recipient to attribute successful outcomes to the expertise of the leader rather than to themselves. More appropriate terminology would be facilitator or coordinator where there is shared decision-making, and success is attributed to the efforts and input of the individual. Teaching the process of learning is therefore critical to self-determination. The true aim of professionals or leaders or indeed parents is to make themselves redundant as the individual realises independence. Issues around the relationship between practitioner and participant in the physical activity context are the subject of Chapter 14.

This is particularly true in our approach to working with older people. A key to lifelong mental well-being is feeling significant, involved and needed, but society is changing in many ways that take away the sense of belonging in older populations. The traditional family structure where grandparents were held in high esteem and had important roles is breaking down. The sense of community and neighbourhood is being lost as amenities and shops are shifting from local to centralised provision. In order to sustain independence, it is already very important to find ways of helping people remain active and valued in society into older age.

Physical activity is an important lubricant for social interaction and helps retain physical and mental function into older age. However, physical activity can also be a very important social agent for all age groups. Children, for example, organise their physical activity around friendship groups (Jago *et al.* 2009). Belonging to clubs or teams whether they involve more traditional sports such as rugby, netball or golf, or activities such as street-dancing squads or informal groups of skateboarders meeting in the park, can be very important for social well-being and developing a sense of social significance.

Physical literacy and the self

The physical self contributes intrinsically through the expression of appearance, physical competence and social engagement in more global aspects of well-being such as self-esteem. It acts as a potent public interface with our world and as such could be regarded as the most powerful element of the self-complex. It is particularly prominent in Western societies where individualism has been entrenched for decades if not centuries. Even in Western societies, historically there have been times when individuality was not accessible to the vast majority of the population who were described by their socio-economic role as serfs or peasants (Baumeister 1987). In collective societies and some spiritual cultures such as Buddhism, the self is less well defined and the physical self is less prominent or even denied. It would seem therefore that the physical self is at least in part culturally determined and the characteristics which make up the physical self will vary from population to population.

Physical literacy is conceptually compatible with the notion of a healthy and positive physical self. A healthy physical self would appear to be one which contributes positively to self-esteem and other elements of psychological well-being such as emotional stability, coping with life demands, life satisfaction and quality of life. It would be oriented towards engagement in healthy behaviours such as physical activity, eating well and positive social interaction. Those who are physically literate and thus could be described as having a healthy physical self would have the capacity to minimise inhibition and overcome lack of confidence to engage, learn and grow. They would display a degree of self-knowledge that recognised strengths and weaknesses, with the maturity to self-accept and work with personal situations in a positive way. Most of all they would have the capacity for healthy adaptation as they progress through the lifecourse.

Physical literacy describes a combination of mental and behavioural attributes that underpin the development and maintenance of a healthy physical self. The concept provides a very useful lens for helping teachers, carers and leaders understand the complex processes involved in facilitating many aspects of well-being throughout the lifecourse.

Recommended reading

Fox, K.R. (1997) The physical self and processes in self-esteem development. In K.R. Fox (ed.) *The Physical Self: From Motivation to Well-being*, Champaign, IL: Human Kinetics (pp. 111–129).

Fox, K.R. (2009) How to help your children become more active. In M. Gonzalez-Gross (ed.) *Active Healthy Living: A Guide for Parents*. Brussels, Coca-Cola Europe (pp. 52–67).

Fox, K.R. and Wilson, P. (2008) Self-perceptual systems and physical activity. In T. Horn (ed.) *Advances in Sport Psychology* (3rd edn), Champaign, IL: Human Kinetics (pp. 49–64).

8 Physical literacy and obesity

Paul Gately

Introduction

It has been argued in Part I that physical literacy can provide a wide range of opportunities in the field of physical activity that can have far-reaching benefits for the quality of life. It is very worrying that the current trend, worldwide, towards obesity is proving to be a serious barrier to many becoming physically literate. These individuals tend to avoid physical activity. Their overall health can suffer, as can their self-confidence and self-esteem. Developing physical literacy can be one way of helping people tackle the problem of obesity. However, as will be seen from the information in this chapter, the situation is far from straightforward. Research has yet to identify clear-cut and proven strategies for the prevention and cure of obesity. While the promotion of physical activity will not in itself provide the remedy, there seems to be growing evidence that interventions which include physical activity programmes can be successful.

This chapter looks at physical literacy in the context of the current problem of obesity in much of the Western world. Causes of obesity are outlined, as are a number of recommendations to tackle the problem. Some of the effects of obesity, particularly in young people, are described. Up-to-date research is drawn on throughout the chapter which concludes with an account of an organised strategy to tackle obesity.

Current levels of obesity

Levels of overweight and obesity have increased significantly in the past three to four decades. It would seem that while the levels and rates of increase vary across the globe, no one country has been immune to increases during this period of time. Table 8.1 presents data from the National Children's Measurement Programme (NCMP) (DoH 2009b) in England, highlighting the high levels of overweight and obesity in children.

These data show that levels of overweight and obesity are high and increase with age. Using these figures it can be estimated that approximately 4.5 million under-18-year-olds in the UK have a weight problem that will

Table 8.1 The percentage of reception and year 6 boys and girls within each weight
category during the National Child Measurement Programme 07/08

	Reception (5 years old)		Year 6 (11 years old)	
	Boys	Girls	Boys	Girls
Obesity	10.4	8.8	20	16.6
Overweight	13.6	12.3	14.4	14.2
Normal weight	74.5	77.9	64.5	67.9
Underweight	1.5	1.0	1.2	1.6

put them at risk of physical and mental health problems. In addition, data
from the Health Survey of England (DoH 2007) (see Figure 8.1) show that
levels of overweight in the adult population have remained relatively stable
during the past fifteen years, while levels of obesity have increased substan-
tially. Such increasing levels of a preventable disease have led to calls for
widespread action from a global to micro level – from the World Health
Organisation and from individuals.

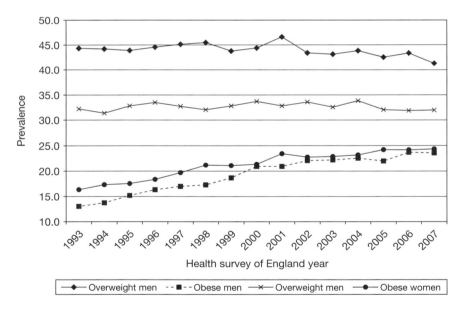

Figure 8.1 Prevalence of overweight and obesity in all men and women 1993–2007.

Obesity is a significant predictor of a range of risk factors for ill-health;
these include: cardiovascular disease, type II diabetes and some forms of
cancer (Flegal *et al.* 2007). With such risks evident in a large number of the

population, the future burden on health services is worrying. A landmark report, *The Foresight Report: Tackling Obesities* (DTI 2007), outlined not simply the health implications of obesity but the broader social and economic impact of this condition. It estimated the annual costs of obesity to the UK economy would reach £50 billion by 2050, with the healthcare costs estimated to be in the region of £10 billion.

Causes and consequences of obesity

The first law of thermodynamics outlines that energy can neither be created nor destroyed, it can only change forms. Thus, weight gain can only be due to a positive energy balance, i.e. if energy intake is greater than energy expenditure. This law is important, since it is the fundamental principle of all weight loss/management advice. While this law is simple and most people can understand its underlying principle, it does not take account of the large number of powerful influences on human energy intake and energy expenditure in the modern world.

While genetic factors are important, genes cannot account for the signifi-cant change in levels of overweight and obesity during the past four to five decades. More relevant are the changes in the environment that have influenced energy intake and energy expenditure. *The Foresight Report* (DTI 2007) outlined a range of physical, psychological, social and cultural factors that have influenced weight gain in the population. A review by Ulijaszek (2007) outlined a number of social and cultural factors which have led to obesity being an inevitable consequence of modern society. According to Hayes *et al.* (2005), dramatic changes in levels of physical activity have occurred from 3.2 PALs prior to efficient tools and machine-based agricul-ture, to 2.2/1.2 PALs in the current population. *The Foresight Report* (DTI 2007: 8) suggested that 'The technological revolution of the 20th century has left in its wake an "obesogenic environment" that serves to expose the biological vulnerability of human beings'.

The increased availability of high-energy dense foods in large portion sizes as well as technological advances that reduce levels of daily physical activity are two of the primary factors which have created this toxic environment. The reduction in physical activity is evident both in respect of labour-saving devices and in the ever-growing range of sedentary leisure pursuits. In addition, inappropriate models given by the media and the growing apprehension on the part of parents to let their children play outside unsupervised exacerbate the situation.

Influence of the media

The relationship between the media and obesity is a significantly under-researched area. The media, including, TV, radio, the internet and magazines has focused heavily on alerting the public to the dangers of becoming overweight and obese. It has supported a range of campaigns that highlight the issue of obesity and in addition has initiated media-style interventions which include some common TV formats/shows such as *Celebrity Fit Club, You are What You Eat* and *The Biggest Loser*. However, the ways in which the media and obesity are associated continues to be unclear, not least because it can itself be a counterproductive influence. For example, the media are prone to promote sedentary behaviours and physical inactivity as well as snacking behaviours. Indeed, some of the earliest research on this issue conducted by Dietz and Gortmaker (1985) showed a positive relationship between TV watching and obesity. Since this study, the outcomes of other similar studies have been inconclusive. Marshall *et al.* (2004: 1238) suggested that: 'Relationships between sedentary behaviour and health are unlikely to be explained using single markers of inactivity, such as TV viewing or video/computer game use.'

Boyce (2007) in a review highlighted the lack of data associated with potential influence on body image. Boyce also commented on the paradox between the scale of the obesity issue and the prominence of the reports associated with underweight. This is supported by Grogan (2008) who reported that within the media, women are portrayed as abnormally slim, while men tend to be portrayed as normal weight. Such messages communicated ubiquitously to a large audience of children and adults are therefore likely to influence the perceptions of overweight and obesity.

Influence of parents

The recent Change4Life public health campaign was underpinned by 'consumer insight' work undertaken by the Department of Health (2008) and provided valuable information about the attitudes and beliefs of parents. Parents were clustered in order to outline specific characteristics which would support guidance on intervention strategies. As covered elsewhere in this book, for example, in Chapter 13, parents are very significant others in influencing young people in respect of exercise participation and physical activity habits.

Some important and relevant insights in the Change4Life campaign included findings such as:

- parents had an inaccurate picture of their weight and the weight of their children;
- many parents had limited awareness of the risks of overweight and obesity;
- parents were often unaware of the association between health and sedentary behaviours;
- parents believed happy children were healthy children;
- parents underestimated their own importance as role models.

More specifically around physical activity issues the following findings were reported:

- children were encouraged and allowed to be sedentary;
- sedentary behaviour was seen as a status symbol;
- children wanted to be active;
- parents believed their children were already active;
- physical activity was a low priority family activity;
- out-of-school activities were seen as too expensive;
- parents were reluctant to exercise themselves;
- playing outside was seen as too dangerous.

These findings are important and demonstrate some of the strong influences arising from family attitudes on physical activity participation. They also clearly demonstrate a culture of physical inactivity being acceptable if not encouraged by the adult population. These insights are not only relevant to children's current and future behaviours, but this research demonstrates the entrenched views of the adult population. Such attitudes need to be addressed as part of strategies to tackle obesity, not least because of the direct influence on parents' behaviours and their own heath and well-being.

The often inaccurate identification of overweight and obesity cited above in respect of parents was also researched by Jeffrey *et al.* (2005). He reported the distorted perceptions of parents about the weight of their overweight and obese children. Jeffry *et al.* found, in 277 parents of children with a range of body weights, that approximately 50 per cent accurately identified their obese child, while only 25 per cent accurately identified their overweight child. Smith *et al.* (2008) conducted a similar study in healthcare professionals and found that approximately 75 per cent of healthcare professionals underestimated overweight children and 50 per cent underestimated the weight category of obese children. These findings were also confirmed in the recent 'Consumer Insight' work conducted by the UK Department of Health as part of the Healthy Weight Healthy Lives strategy (DoH 2008). Given that levels of overweight and obesity have increased significantly over the past four to five decades, as was indicated at the start of the chapter, it may be surprising that perceptions are so flawed. However, these increases are generally associated with approximately 2lb per year weight gain and so the change is somewhat difficult to assess through simple observation.

Prevention and treatment of obesity

Unfortunately the evidence base on the prevention and treatment of obesity is limited. A number of systematic reviews have provided similar conclusions (Epstein and Myers 1998; Summerbell *et al.* 2003), namely that the evidence base on which to draw conclusions is too weak to provide definitive guidance. The National Institute of Health and Clinical Excellence (NICE)

(2006) guidance provides the most pragmatic recommendations for public health workers involved in the delivery of adult and children's obesity interventions. The primary points of this guidance include promoting:

- a supportive and motivating environment;
- family involvement;
- behaviour modification, e.g. goal setting;
- dietary education and advice;
- reduced sedentary behaviours;
- regular lifestyle activity;
- regular structured physical activity/exercise;
- delivery by trained professionals;
- provision of long-term support.

The above list covers a wide range of interventions. While physical activity is important, the evidence base on physical activity as the sole tool to induce weight loss demonstrates that physical activity per se has limited impact on body mass (Epstein and Myers 1998; Summerbell *et al.* 2003). Nevertheless, there have been a number of studies that have looked into forms of physical activity promotion that have been used in obesity interventions for children.

In respect of the physical activity components of obesity, studies have used aerobic exercise in the form of walking, jogging or cycling (Sasaki *et al.* 1987; Epstein *et al.* 1994; Epstein and Goldfield 1999; Gutin *et al.* 1999; Sothern *et al.* 2000). Sasaki *et al.* (1987) used running at lactate threshold which was adjusted monthly to ensure a consistent relative level of exercise intensity. Some studies used sports and games-based activities, but the aim was still to maintain a high-energy expenditure during these sessions (Rocchini *et al.* 1988) Treuth *et al.* (1998) and Sothern *et al.* (2000) reported the use of a resistance training programme. A study by Lee *et al.* (1994) comprised a five-month basic military training programme with overweight and obese Singaporean males aged 17 to 19 years. These provide examples of those researchers who have taken a reductionist approach to physical activity promotion and have specifically prescribed physical activity in the form of designated intensities, frequencies and duration. Such studies may be useful for understanding physiological mechanisms, but they are unlikely to lead to long-term participation in physical activity.

Epstein *et al.* (1994) have provided strong evidence of the benefits of reducing sedentary behaviours, such as limiting access to TV and computer games, rather than promoting specific forms of physical activity. Esptein *et al.* showed significant differences in those children who had been encouraged to reduce their sedentary behaviours compared to those who were prescribed aerobic exercise or calisthenics. The physical activity in this study was structured in the form of cycling on an exercise bike or exercising to an exercise video in a laboratory. Given that such forms of exercise are unlikely to engage children and young people beyond the structured programme, it should not be a surprise to find that the outcomes of the prescribed exercise were limited at long-term follow-up.

Several researchers have developed and assessed a range of alternative forms of physical activity prescription (Cohen *et al.* 1991; Gately *et al.* 2000a). Cohen *et al.* (1991) reported the use of game-type activities such as tumbling, juggling and various ball games. Gately and Cooke (2003a) reported the use of a skill-based fun-type exercise programme and also described the components of their weight management approach, particularly the use of a multicomponent methodology incorporating dietary modification, dietary advice, physical activity and behaviour change.

Considering the range of interventions outlined above, the enhancement of the motivation, confidence and physical competence elements of physical literacy would be more likely outcomes from the interventions that have provided a broad range of experiences, and sought to enthuse and engage young people rather than those interventions that have been more prescriptive and taken a reductionist approach. One of the limitations of the research is the lack of specific outcomes and long-term follow-up (Epstein and Myers 1998; Summerbell *et al.* 2003; NICE 2006). Another of the challenges associated with the evidence base is that very few interventions provide details about the mechanics of these programmes.

The past ten years has seen a major shift in policy development concerned with lifestyle issues to address the challenge of obesity, the focus being primarily associated with preventative strategies to increase physical activity and reduce energy intake. For example, while the Department for Children, Schools and Families policy, Every Child Matters (DfES 2003), is not specifically focused on addressing obesity, its primary objectives should positively influence the precursors of this condition. This has been followed by Choosing Health (DoH 2004b) and more recently *The Foresight Report* (DTI 2007), which outlined not just the health consequences of obesity, but the range of factors which contribute to the issue as well as the financial consequences of obesity. The government response to *The Foresight Report* was the *Healthy Weight Healthy Lives* strategy (DoH 2008) which was supported by a range of further documents. This cross-government strategy is focused on a range of activities to tackle the public health issue of obesity.

The physical consequences of obesity

As indicated in the above data, there are a number of negative consequences associated with obesity. Of particular relevance to physical literacy is a range of research that highlights the impact of being overweight or obese on the physical competences of children or young people. These relate to exercise tolerance, fundamental motor skill development, danger of injury and of cardiovascular problems.

Gately and Cooke (2003b) compared the exercise tolerance of overweight and normal weight children and found significantly lower levels of exercise tolerance in the overweight and obese compared to their normal weight peers, such that the obese children had a 40 per cent lower peak VO_2 than their normal weight peers. Described another way, when the obese child was exercising at an intensity they described as 'very hard', the normal weight child described the same intensity as 'light to moderate'.[1]

Several researchers have shown that fundamental movement skills are strongly associated with physical activity participation (Okely *et al.* 2001; Wrotniak *et al.* 2006; Barnett *et al.* 2008a). These researchers used a number of different definitions (fundamental movement skills, Okely *et al.*; perceived sports competence, Barnett *et al.*; motor proficiency, Wrotniak *et al.*); however, their findings were consistent. Barnett *et al.* (2008b) progressed this research further by investigating the association between motor skill proficiency and adolescent fitness. This study found that children with good object control skills are likely to become fit adolescents. Okely *et al.* (2004) also showed a strong inverse relationship between fundamental movement skills and degree of overweight in both boys and girls. Deforche *et al.* (2008) revealed limited capacity of the overweight and obese compared to their normal weight peers on several static and dynamic balance and postural capacities.

These physical challenges faced by the overweight and obese demonstrate limited physical ability which will hamper current and future levels of physical activity and also contribute to a greater risk of future weight gain.

A further consequence of these physical challenges is the associated perceptions which overweight and obese children have of themselves. Deforche *et al.* (2006) reported a survey of normal weight, overweight and obese children which investigated the benefits associated with participation in physical activity. This study showed that normal weight children rated 'pleasures' as a benefit of physical activity participation significantly higher than their overweight and obese peers. The overweight and obese perceived benefits of 'looking better' and 'losing weight' as significantly more beneficial compared to their normal weight peers. These statements demonstrate a difference in perceived benefits between normal weight children and their overweight/obese peers. These differences may also be described as representing intrinsic motives (pleasure) compared to extrinsic motives (looking better and losing weight). Deci and Ryan (1985) suggest that intrinsic motivation is a strong determinant of future behaviours, indicating clearly that these perceptions are important for future activity levels. This view is very much in line with the view that intrinsic motivation is a key attribute of physical literacy. This motivation is a powerful driver in respect of participating in physical activity, thus enabling individuals to embark on and sustain their personal journey to become physically literate.

With regard to injury, Spaine and Bollen (1996) reported that the mean BMI of adult patients with displaced fractures was significantly higher than those with undisplaced fractures. This was supported by Böstman (1995) who reported data on 3061 patients who presented with a fracture of the distal tibia and ankle. He concluded that being overweight should be recognised as a significant factor in predicting a complicated course after fracture of the lower leg.

A concern that many practitioners have is the risk to the overweight and obese of cardiovascular problems. While this seems a logical concern, the scientific evidence does not support this. A joint position paper between the American Heart Association and the American College of Sports Medicine (AHA/ACSM) (2007) outlined that among young (under 30 years) individuals, the most frequent pathological findings are associated with hereditary or congenital abnormalities. They conclude that the evidence would suggest that the benefits of regular physical activity outweigh the potential risks in respect of overweight and obese individuals.

The psycho-social consequences of obesity

It is very alarming to realise the range and extent of negative psycho-social consequences of obesity. Obese individuals suffer significant prejudice and discrimination. This prejudice has been observed in children as young as 6 years old. Staffieri (1967) showed that children identify silhouettes of obese children as 'lazy, dirty, stupid, ugly, cheats and liars'. Sonne-Holm and Sorenson (1986) identified that social class is influenced by obesity. They found that independent of parental social class, intelligence and education, the obese adult attained a lower social class than comparable normal weight individuals.

Hebl *et al.* (2008) conducted an interesting study into the perceptions of obesity across the lifecourse. They found that younger obese individuals were denigrated to a larger degree than older obese individuals. This demonstrates the greater degree of stigma at a younger age for the obese. Latner *et al.* (2005) in a study of university students reported a high degree of stigmatisation of obesity. Interestingly, participants' weight did not affect their stigmatisation of obesity, with the overweight or obese having similar levels of stigmatising of obesity compared to the non-overweight participants. Friedman *et al.* (2004) furthered this research by investigating the relationship between weight stigmatisation and psychological functioning. They showed that weight-related stigmatisation was predictive of psychological variables, including depression, self-esteem, body image and general psychiatric functioning.

Studies often report that the quality of life of the obese is lower. Schwimmer *et al.* (2003) in a study of paediatric hospital patients outlined significantly lower health-related quality of life. The author reported that as a group they were indistinguishable from children with cancer. A study by Friedlander *et al.* (2003) also reported the association between overweight and obesity and quality of life in a community sample of children. These data are supported by evidence from Walker *et al.* (2003). They showed that in comparison to normal weight peers the overweight and obese had lower levels of global self-worth, perceived athletic competence and appearance. In addition, a study by Hill and Murphy (2000) investigated the levels of self-esteem of obese children characterised by those children who have been teased or bullied for their weight compared to those who have not. These data showed that those obese children who had not been teased or bullied for their weight had similar levels of self-esteem to their normal weight peers. However, those children who were teased or bullied for their weight had significantly lower levels of global self-worth and the domains (school life, social life, athletic ability, appearance and behaviour) compared to their non-teased or bullied obese peers.

Miller *et al.* (2006) found differences in the social behaviours of obese and non-obese adult women, suggesting that these behaviours negatively affect the impressions formed by those with whom they interact. Such social skills may have some influence on children's ability to engage with their peers generally but also on opportunities for physical activity. While exclusion is often considered to be an outcome of obesity, it may also be true that limited social skills exclude a child who then becomes susceptible to future weight gain. This demonstrates the importance of engagement of the overweight and obese child or young person, if such skills are lacking.

Dietz (1998) has provided a summary of consequences of childhood obesity. These include situations in which the obese child:

- was ranked by other children as less likeable;
- experienced decreased acceptance rates for college;
- was less desirable to employers;
- attained a lower level of social class;
- was frequently teased by peers and thus chose younger children as friends;
- had difficulty finding clothes;
- suffered from others overestimating his or her age and expecting more adult behaviour;
- experienced a disturbed body image.

These consequences show the multidimensional challenge of obesity on the social development of the overweight and obese child. The lack of self-esteem, self-confidence and problems interacting with others identified above would seem to support the contention that not being physically literate has a detrimental effect on these aspects of the self. These observations are very much in line with the findings discussed in Chapter 7 on the physical self and physical literacy.

Establishing positive attitudes towards physical activity

In the context of understanding the barriers and benefits of fostering physical literacy in overweight and obese young people it is valuable to look in a little more detail at the importance of physical activity and the significance of the attitudes of young people that affect the establishment of good exercise habits. Physical competence is a key element of physical literacy, as is the motivation to take part in physical activity. This section will consider briefly a range of variables that could support improved exercise habits. The importance of enjoyment and self-efficacy is highlighted.

Total daily energy expenditure consists of:

- basal metabolic rate – the energy used for basic body functioning such as breathing and circulation;
- the thermic effect of food – the energy used during the processes of digestion and absorption;
- spontaneous physical activity – the energy used during fidgeting, which is not under conscious control;
- unrestricted physical activity – the energy used during daily physical activity.

Physical activity is the most variable component of energy expenditure as it is the only aspect under conscious control. It is therefore clear to see why it has been adopted as a component to treat overweight and obesity. Indeed, exercise or physical activity is promoted within a range of guidelines for the prevention and treatment of overweight and obesity (WHO 1997a; NIH 1998). Exercise has been suggested to have favourable effects on a range of anthropometric, body composition, physiological, metabolic and health-related variables including psycho-social health (Blair and Brodney 1999; Ross and Janssen 1999; Rissanen and Fogelholm 1999). In addition, there have been a number of review articles that have demonstrated greater success with the inclusion of exercise in the treatment of overweight and obese children (Bar-Or and Baranowski 1994; Epstein *et al.* 1996; Epstein and Myers 1998; Epstein and Goldfield 1999; Jelalian 1999). Thus, when considering the key ingredients of successful weight management interventions, adherence to physical activity must be a primary objective.

In working to establish good exercise habits it is essential to take seriously the perceptions of young people. Indeed, when considering the important components of weight management programmes for overweight and obese children, Fox (1988) suggests that considering the child's perceptions may be more important than the reality, as children's perceptions will ultimately determine participation. Wankel and Kreisel (1985) suggested that augmenting these perceptions as much as possible within an exercise programme would help to present the programme as a leisure experience and not just as an exercise workout.

Fox (1988) suggested a range of factors that influence participation in physical activity. Important here is that during the development of intervention programmes consideration should be given to the children's experience of the activities and the promotion of adherence rather than simply the anticipated health gains. Fox suggested that children and particularly girls 'perceive that the benefits of taking part do not warrant suffering the inconvenience, discomfort, or feelings of embarrassment or failure that may accompany it' (Fox 1988: 35). This point would be highly relevant to overweight and obese children, who face a range of physical, social, cultural and psychological challenges.

Studies have been conducted to identify reasons for participation in physical activity. Gould (1984) suggested that children's primary reason for participation in exercise is 'to have fun' followed by 'improve skills and learn new skills'. Stucky-Ropp and Dilorenzo (1993) reported in order of importance that boys rated: enjoyment of physical activity, friend and family modelling/support, mothers perceived barriers to physical activity, mothers perceived family support for physical activity as significant predictors of participation. For girls, significant predictors of participation were: enjoyment of physical activity, number of exercise-related items at home, mothers perceived family support for physical activity, mothers perceived barriers to exercise and direct parental modelling of physical activity. Further work by Wankel and Kreisel (1985) provided information on the important aspects of continued physical activity participation; these include competition, curiosity, development of recreational skills, going out with friends and the provision of a range of activities.

Fun and enjoyment are commonly reported as important determinants of physical activity in children (Parker 1991; Sallis and Owen 1997). Strategies that aim to provide an environment that stimulates fun-type exercise and physical activity should therefore be an important element of any intervention programme. Parker (1991) identified that during the development of intervention studies, particularly for overweight and obese children, fun must be a major component to engage children in lifelong physical activity. Bar-Or and Baranowski (1994) suggested that fun-type activities are the best means to enthuse children to exercise and reduce body mass. Wankel and Kreisel (1985) found that across a range of sports the responses relating to enjoyment were extremely consistent. Intrinsic factors such as: excitement of participating in the sport, personal accomplishment, improving one's skills, testing one's skills against others and just doing skills were consistently more important than extrinsic factors such as: pleasing others, receiving rewards or indeed winning the game.

As well as enjoyment, young people need to experience the satisfaction of some improvement in their movement competence. Experience of success is vital for the development of intrinsic motivation. Bandura (1982) proposed that all behaviour changes are mediated by a cognitive mechanism termed self-efficacy. Bandura proposed that 'self efficacy judgements, whether accurate or faulty influence choice of activities and environmental settings. People avoid activities that they believe exceed their coping capabilities, but they undertake and perform assuredly those that they judge themselves capable of managing' (Bandura 1982: 123). Furthermore Sallis and Owen

(1997: 117) suggested that 'Bandura's theory has been strongly supported, because self-efficacy is the strongest correlate of physical activity in virtually every study that it includes'.

One of the primary components of self-efficacy is competence. Harter (1978) proposed that individuals with high perceived physical competence are more likely to participate in physical activity or sport. This is supported by the evidence of Wankel and Kreisel (1985) who showed that competence is an important factor in sports participation, with common responses to the motives for participation in physical activity and sport that included: 'improving one's skills, testing one's skills against others and just doing skills'. Several other authors have proposed competence to be important for children engaging in healthy behaviours (White 1959; Deci and Ryan 1985). This is very much in line with those aspects of the concept of physical literacy that identify motivation, confidence and physical competence as key attributes to this disposition.

Deci and Ryan (1985) have advanced the work of White and others by identifying that competence is a foundation of intrinsic motivation. Deci and Ryan added two further dimensions, which are the need to be self-determining and to be autonomous. Deci and Ryan have proposed that the continuum of extrinsic to intrinsic motivation has a number of elements that are important in engaging children in positive and healthy behaviours. Thus, as was also discussed in Chapter 4, where programmes or interventions are successful in promoting intrinsic motivation in respect of certain behaviours, young people are more likely to adhere to these behaviours.

This suggests that programmes or interventions that concentrate on achieving mastery, developing intrinsic motivation without the need for external recognition (such as rewards) and without the discouraging feelings of being under pressure when performing in the company of peers or significant others are likely to encourage children to engage in long-term physical activity. These findings are very much in line with recommendations made in Chapter 14 which is concerned with learning and teaching approaches that are recommended to foster physical literacy.

Weight loss camp programme

Gately and Cooke (2003a) and Gately *et al.* (2000a, 2000b and 2005) and 2005) have reported the outcomes of two residential weight loss camp programmes for overweight and obese children in North America and the North of England. The programme has used an action research methodology to ensure continued development of the programme. Through quantitative, qualitative and process evaluation research the programme has both developed as well as contributed to the evidence base. This eight-week multidisciplinary residential weight loss programme for children aged 8 to 17 has used the Self Determination Theory approach proposed by Deci and Ryan (1985) as an underlying framework, with a range of social cognitive tools to support the behaviour change of the participants. In addition, physical activity, dietary change and social skill development were essential elements of the intervention.

Gately *et al.* (2005) reported outcomes of children's perceived and actual improvements in sports performance skills. The data showed significant improvements in skills such as basketball shot and badminton serve. This, aligned to significant improvements in perceived athletic competence, demonstrates the holistic impact on overweight and obese attendees of this residential programme. Fitness improvements have also been reported with an average improvement of 18 per cent in the aerobic fitness of overweight and obese participants.

The case study below, telling the story of one camp participant, shows how being motivated to be physically active and being respected by others can have a significant effect on an individual's self-esteem and self-confidence. There is no doubt that Helena grew in physical literacy through her experiences on the camp and that this has brought with it a range of benefits.

Case study 8.1 Helena

Through the help of her GP and support from her Primary Care Trust, Helena was funded to attend the Carnegie International Camp, a residential weight loss camp run by Carnegie Weight Management. Helena, aged 13, had battled with her weight for years (BMI of 31 kg/m) and although she and her family had tried a variety of programmes to lose weight, all results were shortlived and Helena would always fall back into the same routine.

Helena's weight was always a problem and it made her very unhappy, she never had many friends, as people 'judged her for her weight before they got to know her'. Having suffered bullying at school, Helena was nervous about going to Carnegie International Camp. She was also worried about the food being like 'rabbit food' and the exercise being gruelling, 'just like school'.

When she arrived, she was surprised at how happy and enthusiastic the staff seemed. The camp was not what she expected; it was much more fun and she enjoyed learning things with people who understood her. The staff also trusted her and, rather than telling her what to do, they helped her to consider the options and consequences of her choices. She grew in confidence as she moved more easily in the sports activities and made loads of friends. Helena felt normal for the first time in her life. She was finding that she was good at things like boxercise. She also performed her favourite song at a talent show and everyone cheered when she thought they might boo her. She started to feel in control and was confident that with the right support from her family she could really sort out her weight this time.

When she returned home, Helena spoke to her parents and sister for days about her experience on camp; she told her friends that she had been to 'Fat Camp' and 'it was cool'. She followed the plans that she had made on camp. These were realistic, so implementing them into everyday life was easy. She joined in PE and for the first time was told by her teacher that she was 'enthusiastic' and 'committed'. She had lost quite a lot of weight at camp but she 'still had loads to lose'. Helena did not find it easy but knew that she had to work at it.

Six months on, Helena had lost more weight and was eating a healthy diet, which included treats 'but only a few'. She was also involved in a performing arts group and 'the dancing was easy and fun' and she joined an after-school club where she did boxercise. Her next plan was to get a part in the school play. She had loads more friends now and they told her that before they really knew her she had seemed like a 'bit of a loner'. She is now much happier, healthier and believes that she can achieve her goals. Six months on, her weight was much lower and her BMI was down to 26kg/m.

Walker *et al.* (2003) undertook a more specific study into the psychological outcomes of this intervention programme and reported improvements in global self-worth, athletic competence, appearance as well as no increase in the salience of worries of children attending the weight loss intervention. McGregor *et al.* (2005) also found that during the residential intervention for overweight and obese children, global self-worth, perceived athletic competence and appearance were significantly increased over the six-week camp programme. McGregor advanced this work and found that participants perceived a high level of mastery climate, with a moderate level of performance climate. Such an environment is considered important to achieve improvements in self-esteem during weight loss (Reinboth and Duda 2004). Further work from this research group continues to demonstrate the outcomes of such a climate and philosophy.

Barton *et al.* (2004) investigated cognitive changes in the camp given the evidence within both the eating disorder literature and the obesity literature of elevated levels of negative thoughts about shape, weight, food and eating in comparison to normal weight adults. The study reported that attendance at a residential camp was associated with change in cognitive content, demonstrated by a reduction in negative and an increase in positive thoughts associated with exercise. A second finding was that, compared to normal weight children, the obese children who attended the camp initially had more negative thoughts and dysfunctional beliefs and fewer positive thoughts. Post-camp, positive thoughts became normalised, while the dysfunctional beliefs did not change. The authors highlight that the resistance of dysfunctional beliefs to change underscores the level of psychological distress experienced by some adolescents with a weight problem, and demonstrates the level of effort required to achieve long-term weight management in children through engagement in physical activity and healthy eating.

Gately and Cooke (2000) and Gately *et al.* (2000a) have also reported long-term outcomes of the residential weight management programme showing that at one and three years after attending the camps 85 per cent and 96 per cent respectively have a lower standardised BMI than when they started the programme. It is not possible, and probably unachievable, to specifically determine the proportionate contributions of each of the components of this programme. That said, it is clear, based on the acute and long-term outcomes, that a programme which focuses on the promotion of a broad range of physical activities, in a climate that is focused on mastery, relatedness, autonomy and competence is effective in engaging overweight and obese children and young people in physical activity.

Conclusion

These findings provide a valuable framework for promoting physical literacy in children. The evidence presented above demonstrates that according to these criteria overweight and obese children would be considered to have lower levels of physical literacy. In particular, the physical, social, psychological and cultural challenges encountered by overweight and obese children clearly show that they are likely to be at a major disadvantage when compared to their normal weight peers. While the information presented above is primarily focused on the early developmental experiences of children and young people, the longevity of these experiences persists into adulthood, which is supported by data that shows low levels of physical activity in adulthood and increasing levels of overweight and obesity (DoH 2007).

Obesity is clearly an important public health issue given the high prevalence and the associated health and well-being challenges. It is now widely acknowledged that obesity is a difficult issue to address with a range of social, cultural, psychological and physical factors contributing to the increased levels of this condition. Physical activity is a critical component which contributes both directly and indirectly to weight change and to health. It would appear that in terms of the definition of physical literacy used in this book, the achievement of this capability in overweight and obese children is limited. However, it is also clear that with appropriate interventions the physical literacy of overweight and obese children can be improved. This improvement can bring benefits of a more robust self-esteem and better social interaction skills as well as overall health benefits. Interventions focused on long-term engagement through the development of competence and autonomy in a climate that promotes mastery and relatedness are clearly showing signs of success and should be further investigated. These findings demonstrate that a significant amount of work is necessary in this area to further understand the importance of physical activity in the overweight and obese child, and how interventions may seek to improve levels of physical literacy.

Recommended reading

Department For Trade and Industry (DTI) (2007) *The Foresight Report: Tackling Obesities*. HMSO, London.

Jelalian, E., Steele, R.G. and Jensen, C.D. (2009) *Issues in Clinical Child Psychology: Handbook of Childhood and Adolescent Obesity*. Springer, New York.

9 Physical literacy and the young child

Patricia Maude

Introduction

The focus of this chapter is on the roots of physical literacy as they develop in the young child. The first part of the chapter is devoted to the growth and maturation of the infant from birth, with particular reference to physical development. This is followed by a section in which consideration is given to the significant contribution of the acquisition, extension and application of movement vocabulary to the enhancement of physical competence, including the involvement of emerging movement capacities. In the final part of the chapter there is a discussion of the importance of play in the life of the young child, with consideration of how these experiences can foster development of a range of attributes of physical literacy.

This chapter provides opportunities to go right to the core of physical literacy in action, as evidenced in young children. Commencing with the embryonic emergence of attributes of the concept at the start of life, even before birth, consideration is given to key aspects of physical literacy in all its richness as infants develop physically, mature and learn through movement experience and exploration of their environment.

The short definition of physical literacy states that:

> *As appropriate to each individual, physical literacy can be described as the motivation, confidence, physical competence, knowledge and understanding to maintain physical activity throughout the lifecourse.*

The full definition of physical literacy embraces not only these attributes, but also aspects of imagination, self-esteem, interaction with the environment and interaction with others. Each of these attributes, when nurtured in early childhood, throughout the waking hours of each day, can provide a firm foundation for a rich and enduring development of physical literacy throughout the lifecourse. Exploring the development of the attributes of physical literacy in the young child constitutes the significant contribution of this chapter to those which precede and follow. For example, it builds from the discussion in Chapter 4 in detailing the rich range of movement patterns on which it has been suggested that the child's concept development and awareness of self are founded. Looking ahead to Chapter 15, the identification of these movement patterns lays the ground for further analysis of the constituents of movement.

The young child in the very short case study below ably demonstrates the emergence of many of the attributes of a physically literate individual. Not only is she seen here to build on her physical competence and movement capacities, but she also reveals her motivation and confidence. She demonstrates independence, an ability to interact with the environment and a level of knowledge and understanding that enables her to make the significant progress that is shown in this illustration. Case study 9.1 is thus

---

Case study 9.1 Emily

Emily, aged 3, was watching the children riding running bikes in the outdoor area at her day nursery. She was usually a shy child. Although she was apparently physically competent, with sound cephalo-caudal development, a mature pattern of locomotion and good coordination, she had not been brave enough to venture outdoors alone or to run around with the other children. She was reluctant to try new activities, including those suggested by her key worker. The first time I observed her, she ventured outdoors to watch other children successfully riding their running bikes, balancing on two wheels, taking their feet off the ground and free-wheeling with joy and exhilaration down the path, then putting their feet down again to stop. She walked over, chose a running bike and patiently found out both how to hold the handlebars to keep the bike upright and to step across it with one foot in order to balance with her feet on the ground in order to sit steadily on the seat. She 'gingerly' walked a few steps forward, followed by more steps until she came to the edge of the play area, where she stopped and worked out how to turn around. The next time I watched her, she too could run a few steps to get going, could take her feet off the ground and, keeping her balance, could feel the freedom of being carried along momentarily, before putting her feet back down to stop.

The brilliant concept of the running bike is that it provides for the key fundamental movement capacity needed in bike riding: that of balancing, upright, on a moving two-wheeler. Without the impediment of also having to concentrate on pedalling, children can find out for themselves, unaided, how to maintain balance while also controlling the handlebars and managing the movement and stopping of the bike. Once these are achieved, away they go, gradually increasing their speed before taking their feet off the ground and also managing to put them back down to stop.

a springboard for the entire chapter, as many of the attributes of a physically literate child are considered in each of the three sections which follow, commencing with the development of physical competence.

Early movement development towards physical competence

The first section of this chapter is devoted to the growth and maturation of the infant from birth. This includes brain development and reveals the crucial importance of physical activity as a stimulus to the development of the brain.

From birth, the brain develops from the base upward, with the lower or sensori-motor area leading the way, through its management of all aspects of basic survival and functioning. The sensori-motor area of the brain enables learning to take place through the senses of touch, sight, sound, taste and smell, and relies on movement to provide the main stimulus. Thus the random movements of the newborn trigger the arousal mechanisms in the brain, as if telling the brain to wake up and make sense of the world around. Later in infancy and early childhood, once the sensori-motor section of the brain has developed, other areas of the brain, such as those controlling automatic movement, rhythm and emotion embark on their maturation. For example, located in the upper part of the brain is the area which controls higher order thinking and other aspects of cognitive development essential for academic achievement. Neglect of attention to ensuring extensive and rich sensori-motor activity can lead to developmental delay and deprivation. Similarly, lack of appropriate sensori-motor activity may lead to delay in the development of the mid-brain, responsible for affective and social activity as referred to in Chapter 6.

At birth, the brain is still underdeveloped, being made up of billions of cells which are not yet connected up. For the essential connections to take place the cells need to be stimulated. Physical activity is the key stimulus to brain development. Ratey and Hagerman (2008) state that physical activity is crucial to brain development and maintenance and is seminal to the way we think and feel. They suggest that there are three ways in which exercise assists brain development: first, by activating that part of the brain that is responsible for alertness, attention and motivation; second, by enabling the efficient working of the billions of active brain cells, and third, by promoting a process called 'neurogenesis', which stimulates the growth of new brain cells. Their research concludes (2008: 4): 'exercise cues the building blocks of learning in the brain' and (2008: 245) is 'the single most powerful tool to optimise brain function'. For optimum brain development infants and children need to be physically active for a significant percentage of their waking hours. Furthermore, they state (2008: 3), 'we are born movers' and suggest that we are 'at peril of dulling the brains of the next generation' if we fail to ensure that every young child continually builds on their physical competence birthright through frequent physically active play. This is supported by Hoeger and Hoeger (1993: 148), who state: 'Movement and physical activity are basic functions for which the human organism was created.' Although we are, in Ratey and Hagerman's terms, 'born movers', the journey towards physical competence in fact commences before birth. As early as the sixth week after conception, the growing foetus may be seen to be moving reflexively and without apparent purpose in the womb. While this may seem like random activity, this movement is preparation for life after birth and is part of an organised movement system that progresses, if used effectively, throughout life. 'Children are born with approximately a hundred reflexes' (Cheatum and Hammond 2000: 59), many of which are necessary for survival, while others must disappear and become integrated into new movement patterns.

The primitive reflexes, stimulated by the brain, that are seen before birth continue to be evident as involuntary movements after birth. These include, for example, the rooting and sucking reflexes, essential for feeding. Another example, the stepping reflex, may be seen in newborn infants when held upright with their feet resting gently on a horizontal surface, make stepping actions. This involuntary reflex activity normally disappears soon after birth. Thereafter, the process of learning to walk as a voluntary action is the result of many progressive activities, in a predictable sequence, with much trial and error, as the child strives to increase strength, balance, posture, core stability, muscle tone, head control and coordination of the limbs. Walking is thus spurred by natural maturation of the musculo-skeletal system, and the development of movement capacities such as coordination and spatial awareness.

Consideration now moves to those aspects of the growth and development of the skeleto-muscular and nervous systems that relate to early aspects of physical competence, enabling young children to capitalise on their genetic inheritance as they grow and mature.

Physical development can be defined as the continuous process through which the child grows and matures from the newborn infant towards the mature adult. This includes growth and the development of the skeleton, muscles, ligaments, tendons, the brain, nervous system and all the internal organs that function without our conscious attention, to keep us alive. All of these body systems need to be continually and actively encouraged to thrive, in order to achieve optimum performance and to support future survival. Between birth and 5 years of age the child experiences a phenomenal range of changes and developments, for example, in shape, size, muscular strength and physical competence. Thus children experience the world as ever-changing, they discover new potentials, realise attainable challenges and fail in unattainable challenges, on an almost daily basis. This restless interaction with the environment was described earlier in Chapter 3 in terms of intentionality which drives individuals to build relationships with the world through perception and response.

Child development follows an organised sequence of developmental stages, with each child progressing through the sequence at a unique personal rate, according to genetic endowment and daily experience. The sequence of developmental stages is normally the same for all children, regardless of culture, though the pace is dependent on 'individual traits, environment and child-rearing practices' (Maude 2001: 7). For example, children with disabilities may progress at a slower pace.

Two principles dictate the sequence of physical development. These are known as 'Cephalo-caudal' and 'Proximo-distal'. Cephalo-caudal growth concerns 'top-downward' development, such that the upper body increases in strength and control before the lower limbs, with the ankles and feet being the last to mature in this sequence. In detail, the early part of the sequence involves gaining strength in the muscles of the neck, which control the movement of the head, in order, for example, to look towards a stimulus. This action precedes those of lifting and holding up the head. This latter activity, when lying on the front, requires management of the shoulders, as in pushing up from front lying, whereby the muscles around the upper back, front and shoulders enable the infant to raise the head and look around, thereby gaining control and increasing strength in the shoulders. Front lying is therefore essential for promoting cephalo-caudal development. Not only does it enable the infant to learn to push up, to raise the head, using the arms, facilitating the strengthening of the upper part of the spine, but it is also essential for strengthening the postural muscles of the middle and lower spine. Muscular strength enables control of the spine and later of the hips so that the sequence of development of locomotion progresses through mastering rolling over, creeping, crawling, sitting with support and later without support. These in turn precede further development of the muscles around the hips, knees and ankles and feet. As the muscles around these joints become more frequently exercised, they increase in strength until the infant is ready for weight-bearing on the feet in order to come to a standing position, first with and then without support, prior to learning to take the first step towards walking and eventually to the achievement of full locomotion. However, as the 'leg end' is the later cephalo-caudal part to develop, young children need to engage in much locomotor activity, not only to strengthen the leg muscles, but to ensure efficient use of the hip, knee and ankle joints. Rather than retaining elements of early reflexive movement they will thereby establish a voluntary pattern of locomotion and readily progress to adding travelling actions such as jogging, running, leaping, galloping, hopping and skipping to their movement vocabulary.

Prior to the 1990s, babies spent many hours in front lying. This was vital movement development time well spent. Since then, however, fears of the 'cot-death' syndrome have led to infants being laid on their backs rather than on their fronts, both to sleep and to play. It has been reported that over 600 hours of 'tummy time' in the first year have thereby been denied to many of this generation of infants. Not only is front lying essential for the development of balance in readiness for upright posture, eye focus and righting of the head, but it also encourages strong and efficient functioning of the heart and lungs through the building up of the chest muscles. A further inhibition to the normal pattern of the development of locomotion has been caused by a recent trend of keeping infants in 'containers', such as beanbags and rigid seats which virtually encase them. Although containers are seen to keep children safe, they can seriously restrict freedom of movement and detrimentally limit the amount of activity necessary to strengthen the postural muscles of the spine and the weight-bearing muscles of the legs in preparation for walking.[1] Those children whose early sensori-motor development has been compromised are more likely to present in later childhood with delayed movement coordination. Children who are unable to move slowly, to come to a stop with control, to sit still when appropriate, who always seem to be 'fussy' and hurried movers may well have retained aspects of involuntary movement. Delay in movement development can also be seen in children whose arms flail out sideways to help them to maintain balance as they run. In the mature running pattern the flexed arms swing forward and back to streamline and add power to the run.

The second principle of development is known as proximo-distal development, whereby controlled movement matures from the more central parts of the body outward, such that the shoulder muscles strengthen before those of the elbows, with the wrist and hand muscles maturing much later. Proximo-distal development can be evidenced when infants flail their arms around, in a random swiping action, initiated from the shoulders, but with no controlled use of the elbows, lower arms, wrists or hands. This apparently indiscriminate, involuntary movement of the arms from the shoulders enables the infant to discover how to bring the hands together at the midline of the body, subsequently discovering the mouth with the hands and later grasping objects and trying to put them into the mouth.

The muscles of the upper and lower arms which control extension and flexion of the elbows mature later than the shoulders. For example, mature movement around the wrist joints cannot be completed until the wrist bones have differentiated from their cartilaginous state at birth. Thereafter the muscles which will control the fine movements of the wrists and hands need much activity in order to gain strength. For this reason young children adopt the palmar or power grip of tools and use the shoulder, rather than the wrist to guide the tool as, for example, in the sweeping and swiping-like actions seen when painting. The fine or tripod grip of the writing tool, needed for successful letter formation, cannot be achieved until the muscles of the wrists into the palms have gained the strength needed to enable the fingers to exert sufficient pressure on the writing tool. Coordinated manipulation of tools and other fine motor activities are dependent upon successful distal development. These are also dependent upon a sufficient and extensive experience of gross motor, or large muscle activity which will be discussed further in the next part of the chapter.

Promotion of effective cephalo-caudal and proximo-distal development is essential both for complete sensori-motor development and for the achievement of physical competence. Promotion of extensive physical activity is also essential for stimulating optimum brain development. As Ratey and Hagerman (2008: 4) say: 'To keep our brains at peak performance, our bodies need to work hard'. Promotion of exercise in the form of extensive gross motor activity, to underpin and enhance effective fine motor activity is paramount for the development of well-coordinated and controlled physical competence. Case study 9.1 illustrates some of the progress Emily had made with regard to these developmental features, particularly in relation to cephalo-caudal and proximo-distal development, gross motor activity and the development of balance.

Development of movement vocabulary, movement memory and movement quality towards physical competence

In relation to all other age-groups in the lifecourse, children in their early years experience the greatest rate of progress in those aspects of physical competence which involve the acquisition of movement vocabulary. Newborn infants arrive with a wealth of movement vocabulary that enables them not only to engage in the primary function of survival, but also to interact with their environment. When laid on their backs, babies are free to kick their legs, wave their arms and turn their heads. Indeed, they can be more active in this supine position than when laid, prone, on their fronts, although the prone position is essential as the basic position from which to develop locomotion, as discussed above. Apart from time spent in sleeping, resting between bouts of movement activity, eating and other essential systems-sustaining functions, young children's lives are normally movement orientated. They seem to be constantly engaged in discovering new movements, often through trial and error, as well as by repeating, practising and refining those movements already experienced.

Three notable features of physically competent movers are the extent of their movement vocabulary, the accuracy and size of their movement memory and the refinement in the quality of their movement. These three elements of movement form the foundation for the development of physical competence which is at the heart of physical literacy. Consideration of these three aspects of physical competence makes up this part of the chapter.

Movement vocabulary can be described as the movement version of the content of a dictionary for speakers. Whereas a dictionary is made up of millions of individual words, the movement vocabulary comprises the millions of movements that are humanly possible. Thus, these myriads of movements are the ingredients of the total movement vocabulary of the mover, just as words are the ingredients of the total verbal vocabulary of the speaker.

Movement vocabulary can be organised into series of categories, rather like the A to Z of a dictionary. For example, the two simple categories of 'gross' and 'fine' muscle activity could be adopted. Movement involving the large muscles, such as in walking, running, climbing, rolling, breast stroke swimming, diving and leaping would fall into the gross group, and manipulative movements, often involving the muscles of the hands as in writing, operating a keyboard, pegging clothes on to a line, cutting, sewing, picking up and setting down toys, would fall into the fine category. However, in order to explore the widest possible range of movement vocabulary, for young children, the following seven categories are presented: balance, locomotion, flight, manipulation, projection, construction and non-verbal communication (see Table 9.1).

Although these examples constitute just a small sample of a young child's movement vocabulary, they are included in order to signal a range of movement categories and to represent some starting points from which further movement vocabulary can be developed.

Other categories could be proposed, for example, according to the mover's location and environments, such as indoors and outdoors, in garden and playground and park, in woods and water, on grass and beach; or according to the resources and equipment available, such as natural, manufactured and self-created.

Movement memory is the internalising of movements experienced. The movement patterns of single actions, initially established as experimental experiences, are gradually refined through practice, repetition and maturation, until they become automatic. At this stage they can be recalled and used as if without having to be thought about in order for them to be performed. For example, movement memory enables all the elements of the two-footed jump to be automatically recalled and executed effectively. In performing single actions such as a two-footed jump, there are three phases, each dependent on the preceding phase for success. These phases may be termed the preparation, the action and the landing. Forward and upward arm swing, coordinated with flexion of the hips, knees and ankles and forward focus of the eyes, precedes successful explosive arm swing and leg joint extension, to project forcefully vertically upwards, in order to descend with control, downward arm swing, flexion of the leg joints, accurate use of the ankles and feet to land on two feet with resilience. Movement memory enables all these elements of the two-footed jump to be automatically recalled and executed effectively. This single action will be practised by most young children as soon as their legs are strong enough to enable them both to push themselves off the ground and also to resist gravity in order to land without falling over. Gradual refinement of the three phases then takes place throughout childhood.

Movement memory is further challenged when performing a series of actions in sequence. Here, the mover must not only recall the single actions which are the individual components of the sequence, but also the linking

Table 9.1 Movement vocabulary: categories and examples

Balance: vocabulary to enhance stable support and postural control									
on front	on back	on side	on bottom	upside-down as in handstand	on hands and feet	on hands and knees	on knees	on feet	on one hand and one foot
on one foot	sliding				on elevated, wide and narrow surfaces				
Locomotion: vocabulary to enhance travel from place to place									
creeping	slithering	crawling	stepping	walking	jogging	running	rolling	skipping	galloping
pulling	pushing	swinging	climbing	swimming			rocking	scooting	biking
Flight: vocabulary to enhance projecting oneself off the ground and back down to land									
landing on two feet	taking off	jumping up		jumping along		jumping onto		jumping off	jumping over
landing on one foot	hopping	hopscotch		leaping		abseiling		jumping with turn	assisted flight
Manipulation									
holding	feeling	grasping	gripping	drawing	tracing	guiding	cutting	pegging	threading
moulding	typing	mouse management	picking up		receiving a rolled object		catching		
Projection									
grasping	releasing	placing	rolling	bouncing	throwing	striking	heading	aiming	kicking
punting	volleying	flicking	flinging	spinning	skimming	serving	goal shooting		
Construction									
picking up	lifting	carrying	arranging	assembling	adjusting	stacking	building	dismantling	storing
Communication (non-verbal)									
pointing	waving	clapping	smiling	frowning	beckoning	bowing	curtsying	turning towards	turning away

movements, or joining actions, which create the link between one component and the next. Developing movement memory is a constant challenge for young children, both in extending their movement vocabulary and in managing sequencing. In Case study 9.1 above, Emily shows both her increasing movement vocabulary and her progress in sequencing as she puts together and repeats the actions necessary to master bike riding. Evidence of progress is also seen daily in mastering routines such as the ordering and management of dressing and undressing, or the efficient sequence of cleaning teeth. As adults, we scarcely consider the components and linking actions in these seemingly automatic sequences and are probably thinking of other matters at the same time. For a learner coming newly to the task, cleaning teeth can be not only a complex series of single actions that need to be linked for successful fulfilment, but also a supreme challenge. This requires ordering and linking of the single actions related to managing the brush, the paste, the water and the brushing actions in the upper and lower jaw to achieve the sequence from start to finish. The movement memory required for linking series of actions is called on throughout childhood and throughout life, both in daily tasks and in specialised activities. For example, in more sophisticated situations such as a gymnastics sequence, made up of a jump, followed by a roll and completed in a balance, the learner must first be able to perform each of the single actions, such as with the jump described above. The sequence involves learning and then anticipating and recalling the links that enable the sequence to progress from one action to the next.

Movement quality is the outcome of embedding elements of the movement vocabulary into the movement memory, so that they can be recalled into action with poise, coordination, efficiency, accuracy and usually with the minimum of effort. Movement quality is the result of refining and honing each element in the movement vocabulary, from crude early trials, through guidance, repetition and maturation until movement mastery and movement memory are achieved. For example, the individual elements of jumping, rolling and balancing, discussed above, will have been within the movement experience and movement vocabulary of most children from an early age, with the movement memory element involving sequencing, developing in later childhood. However, movement quality is also dependent upon application and incorporation of movement capacities such as coordination, orientation in space, dexterity, precision, fluency and rhythm. Movement capacities develop incrementally throughout childhood, as the child gains experience, but they are also dependent upon the individual's growth patterns and maturation rates, as these will determine, for example, muscular strength, power and stamina. Each component of the gymnastic sequence, along with the linking movements that join them, is also enhanced as the young child develops other movement capacities such as balance, coordination, ability to move with varying speeds and ability to determine accurate placement of the limbs and spine. This serves as an example of ways in which physical literacy is enhanced through developing physical competence elements of movement vocabulary, movement memory, movement quality and movement capacities.

Maturation also plays a key role as the child grows and can be a significant hurdle in young children where physical immaturity temporarily inhibits attainment of aspects of physical literacy. For example, during the first two years, the eyes are developing rapidly, facilitating increased clarity of vision, ability to focus, to track objects and to judge distance However, it is not until about the age of 4 that the eyes have normally matured sufficiently for the child to be able to distinguish an oncoming object from its background, as is essential for catching a ball. Eye maturation is crucial to success. Even if the child has learnt to move the feet to the path of the ball, to prepare the hands for the catching action and can watch the ball, unless the eyes are able to determine the location, speed and power of the oncoming missile and to distinguish the ball from the background, then success is in jeopardy. For example, again considering the catching action, there are many progressions that can precede catching a thrown ball that are appropriate as the child matures. These include grasping a ball from the hands of the sender, passing the ball from hand to hand or around the body, gently rolling a ball and retrieving it, sitting, then standing to receive into the hands a ball rolled along the ground, catching a ball as it rises from a bounce, catching from an underarm throw and catching from an overarm throw. Add to these the multiplicity of shapes, textures and dimensions of missiles such as beanbags, balloon balls, large, medium and small foam balls and the opportunities for enhancing movement quality are endless. The role of parents and significant others is crucial in guiding children's learning and through providing appropriate experiences. The important role of parents in encouraging and facilitating physical competence and thus ensuring a sound springboard for the development of physical literacy has already been mentioned in Chapter 7 and will be picked up again in Chapters 13 and 14. Helping children to achieve movement quality depends not only upon our knowledge of developmental factors such as those described above, but also upon consideration of the many progressive stages that lead to movement mastery. Seefeldt (1993) states that children who have been deprived or frustrated in their early movement experience often avoid physical activity and thereby develop inadequate movement skills. They may then go on to feel excluded from the play experiences enjoyed by their peers and this may eventually lead to a lifetime of inactivity.

Appropriate, individualised provision for children with delayed movement development and children with disabilities is of paramount importance if they are to access the richest movement experience available and to achieve their potential in physical literacy. This is considered in further depth in Chapter 11. Early childhood is the breeding ground for the physical competence attribute of physical literacy. Movement vocabulary, movement memory and movement quality are essential components of the physically competent person. Where young children have successfully embarked on the acquisition of these components, these can then be continually applied, adapted and refined in the wide range of movement tasks undertaken throughout life.

Play and physical literacy

For the young child, the business of life is experienced through play and, to this end, the final part of this chapter is devoted to consideration of some of the key features of play and opportunities thereby for enhancing physical literacy. The activities of play and the opportunities offered through play determine the richness of daily life for all young children, including those with disabilities. Chapter 11 is concerned with promoting physical literacy in those with a disability, and endorses the importance of access to a wide range of physical activity opportunities for these individuals. Play both nurtures the child's emergent physical literacy and is the major vehicle for early learning. Early movement development, discussed in the first part of the chapter, and increase in movement vocabulary, movement memory and movement quality, discussed in the second part, are dependent upon a rich and extensive play experience. Indeed, the development of the physical competence attribute of physical literacy is reliant upon play. Singer (2006) suggests that play provides for creativity and spontaneity, it poses problem-solving opportunities and promotes intellectual growth. Play also facilitates the establishment of many of the other attributes that are characteristic of a physically literate individual, including motivation, confidence, environ-mental and interpersonal engagement, self-knowledge and self-expression. The case study of Emily ably demonstrates a number of benefits that she was gaining through her play, including venturing outdoors alone, tackling a new and challenging task, learning to balance and to take risks. She also appeared to be considerably increasing her self-confidence. Children's burgeoning physical literacy can be further enhanced through play by the access afforded by a wide range of resources and environments, particularly the outdoors, and by interaction with other children and adults who engage alongside and with the child at play.

Play has been defined (Play England 2006: 2) as 'freely chosen, self-determined and without adult intervention'. This approach to play may be defined as 'free' play. The proponents of this interpretation suggest that through the provision of play places where children feel safe, with appro-priate equipment and resources, they will naturally become physically competent. Free play enables children to engage at will, to capitalise on their natural abilities to be imaginative and to follow their own initiative. However, free play alone is not sufficient for children to gain these benefits or achieve their potential in terms of physical literacy. Even children who are naturally active, energetic and inquisitive, physically competent, wide-ranging and self-challenging in their play will nevertheless be constrained by the limitation of their own experience. Furthermore, children who neither choose to play outdoors nor to engage in energetic gross movement play, who do not use their initiative to explore their environment and the resources within it, will be even more severely deprived in developing physical competence and other attributes of physical literacy. Using the analogy of language vocabulary and reading, it is not normally expected that children will learn to read simply by releasing them into an environment full of word resources and books. Neither ought we to expect physical competence, including articulate, poised, efficient and expressive movement just to emerge through free play. The young child's learning through play needs to be supported by the knowledgeable involvement of adults. Through the guidance and encouragement of parents and carers promoting, enriching and nurturing physical competence, young children can 'move outside the box' of their own experience and extend their physical literacy immeasurably and to great effect.

A sufficient play experience is best achieved through a mixture of free play, guided play and play in formal settings through to involvement in structured play. Guided play, involving parents and other adults, can provide a powerful enhancement both to physical competence and to all-round development and learning. For example, a child repeatedly trying and failing to hit a ball towards a target can be helped to success by bringing the target nearer, by pushing the ball along the ground, by modelling the activity, shown by an adult, or by the adult guiding the child's batting hand. Helping a child who wants to skip can be achieved by playing hopping games and walking and hopping games together, hand in hand and by slowly stepping and hopping side by side and towards each other. Young children thereby can be encouraged to explore ever-increasing opportunities afforded by their play environment, can gain greater experience of the natural resources around them and take fuller advantage of the equipment put at their disposal. Structured play, with intended outcomes that are planned to meet children's learning needs, not only adds richness to their experience but can also ensure that they gain the widest range of experience. For example, The Early Years Foundation Stage in England (DCSF 2007) provides a resource of planned learning experiences for children around six areas of learning, one of which is Physical Development. Maude (2008) suggests some aims and content of a Physical Development programme.

Vygotsky (in Singer 2006) suggests that the act of play extends far beyond the recreational factor. Play enables children to learn many skills beyond physical competence, such as decision-making, turn-taking, language, social skills, interaction, monitoring and reciprocity. The example in Case study 9.2 illustrates this well. The context of this case study is a nursery school in England. An increasing number of nurseries in this country and abroad, particularly in Scandinavian countries, build the curriculum on the Forest Schools approach, which offers children a daily programme of free play, guided play and structured play through outdoor experience. The objectives of this approach are to develop children's physical competence, language and communications skills, social skills, including team working, knowledge and understanding of the environment, self-confidence and self-belief and increased motivation and concentration. In addition, children learn about safety, risk management and personal decision-making.

Perry (2001: 118) suggests that 'Outdoor play settings may be the one place where children can independently orchestrate their own negotiations with the physical and social environment and gain the clarity of selfhood necessary to navigate later in life.' Outdoor play also engages children in physical learning through exploratory experiences which engage them meaningfully, purposefully and with imagination in more extensive and natural environments than can normally be provided indoors. If we add to these the benefits to be gained in terms of exercise, creative, cognitive, spatial and communication development as well as opportunities to become risk literate and physically literate, we are presented with overwhelming evidence for the benefits of outdoor play for young children.

Case study 9.2 YMCA Fairthorne Manor Day Nursery

A visit to YMCA Fairthorne Manor Day Nursery (www.ymca-fg.org) revealed the effectiveness of this approach. Having walked some way away from the nursery building, out across a stream and into the woods, we found the children playing freely in what seemed like a huge unfenced forest area. At first the children were playing freely, fully absorbed in mixing sand and soil, making hiding places, seemingly away from adult gaze, digging tiny holes near the roots of huge forest trees with minute trowels, finding treasures andrunning hither and yon on important and private matters. Their teachers, play leaders and carers were both non-participant and participant. They both observed the children and guided them in their play. Sometimes an adult became a playmate for a while and at other times would demonstrate and model an activity in order to encourage and extend a child's experience. In addition to the free and guided play, the morning included a session of structured play. This 'Sounds' session had been preplanned, with a large selection of resources in the form of 'boom-whackers' (tuned plastic pipes), already set out and adults ready to introduce the activity. Watching a group of 3-year-olds experiencing sounds in the woods was a revelation. The adults encouraged the children to keep still and listen to the natural sounds and rhythms around them, to the sounds out in the open and from near a tree, including birds, the feet of others and the sounds coming from the outdoor fireplace. Then the children went running through the woods with their boomwhackers, listening to the sounds they produced and to the volume of their boomwhackers and to the sounds made by those of other children near and far. From that morning's activity the children experienced freedom of movement to explore large outdoor spaces and to develop their physical competence, listening skills and spatial awareness, in a situation where constraints on volume of sound and extent of space to explore seemed almost unlimited. The children also had opportunities to develop their language and vocabulary, in relation not only to sound but also to concepts of space, speed and size.

Following this structured play activity the children either carried on with sound play or found other exciting and absorbing activities. The adults continued observing, guiding and extending the children's experiences.

The blend of free play and adult-involved guided play and adult-planned structured play, as detailed in Case study 9.2, enabled the children both to rely on and build upon their own resources and to be further stimulated into new experiences by their teachers, carers and play-leaders. Through guided and structured play children's creative play and spontaneous activity can be enhanced, while also providing for increased problem-solving opportunities and stimulation of intellectual growth. In addition to praise, encouragement and guidance, there are many other functions that significant others can undertake in supporting the enhancement of physical competence in young children. These include demonstrating, or modelling, through movement and language, as well as facilitating social development and nurturing move-ment imagination and creative development. Parents and carers can join in as playmates or as models of good practice to help scaffold children's learning. They can also raise expectations, show how to take safe risks, and present safe and attainable challenges. Through positive and developmental feedback parents and carers can nurture confidence and self-motivation. Through modelling physical activity they can increase a young child's move-ment vocabulary, extend movement sequencing and demonstrate movement quality in building physical competence.

Conclusion

Enabling young children to increase their movement vocabulary, movement memory and movement quality is fundamental to building their physical competence. Play environments, both indoors and outdoors, play resources, both natural and manufactured, playmates, both adults and children, are key to the promotion of physical literacy. Play can provide a rich context for the nurturing of physical literacy, offering a wealth of opportunities for new experiences and challenges and for enhanced growth and development.

Embarking on the physical literacy journey is at the heart of early childhood development, wherein the infant can capitalise on the experiences encountered from birth, to build upon the unique abilities with which they were born. Ensuring that young children achieve their physical literacy potential is a rich investment in lifecourse achievement.

Recommended reading

Cheatum, A. and Hammond, A. (2000) *Physical Activities for Improving Children's Learning and Behaviour: A Guide to Sensory Motor Development.* Human Kinetics, Champaign, Ill.

Maude, P. (2001) *Physical Children Active Teaching.* Open University Press, Buckingham.

Maude, P. and Whitehead, M.E. (2003) *Observing Children Moving.* CDRom, afPE.

Ratey, J.J. and Hagerman, E. (2008) *SPARK: The Revolutionary New Science of Exercise and the Brain.* Little, Brown & Company, New York.

10 Physical literacy and the older adult population

Len Almond

Introduction

This chapter explores the relevance of physical literacy as a lifespan issue with a particular focus on older adults to illustrate the argument. Issues addressed in the chapter include a range of problems associated with the lack of physical activity in the lives of older adults, the reluctance to enjoy being active on a regular basis and some of the reasons for this state of affairs. The discussion will then consider the concept of physical literacy in respect of the adult population and present a case for the promotion of physical literacy as an essential goal in lifelong education. The chapter concludes by bringing together all aspects of the arguments to demonstrate their relationships and to propose an integrated approach to the promotion of physical literacy.

The promotion of physical activity is often justified on the grounds that it can reduce the risks of people acquiring specific medical conditions or delay the onset of functional decline. This prevention agenda also sees physical activity as a way of reducing the costs of ill-health. This argument appears to have little power in persuading people to become more active and therefore a different more positive perspective needs to be adopted. This situation provides the background to exploring a personal perspective to physical literacy and identifying two additional factors that it is valuable to consider in the development of this capability and its role in influencing the lives of young and old. As an outcome of this position it is pertinent to explore physical literacy as a goal throughout the lifecourse together with a concept called a pedagogy of engagement.

Background

A significant body of compelling scientific evidence (DoH 2004a, 2008; USDHHS 2008) indicates that regular physical activity can bring significant health benefits to people of all ages and abilities. If one looks at the Health Survey for England (DoH 2007) it is quite clear that very few people, especially adults beyond 45 years, value exercise, the figures being so low. Over 70 per cent of adults do not take part in sufficient exercise to meet national guidelines. By the age of 75 only 9 per cent of men and 4 per cent of women are doing 30 minutes of physical activity on at least five days per week. Table 10.1 illustrates how little exercise older adults undertake.

Table 10.1 Percentage of people who do not do sufficient physical activity to benefit their health (%)

	Men	Women
45–55 years	62	66
55–64 years	65	73
65–74 years	79	84
75+	92	96

Source: Health and Social Care Information Centre (HSCIC) (2009).

The costs of inactivity to the health service are substantial, yet only a small proportion of people who are inactive can claim that their medical condition limits their participation in physical activity. In other words, much of the health costs are caused by lifestyle choices, a lack of commitment to regular physical activity or a lack of awareness of the importance of being active.

In addition, people over the age of 50 represent the most sedentary segment of the adult population (Sport England 2006a). Sedentary behaviour such as long spells of sitting, that is, sitting for two hours or more, is seen as a risk factor for a number of medical problems (Hamilton *et al.* 2008; Owen *et al.* 2009) and low levels of physical activity contribute significantly to a major decline in functional capacity among older people, which in turn can lead to limitations in everyday life. For older adults, muscle mass and strength, endurance, bone density and flexibility are all 'lost' at a rate of about 10 per cent per decade after the age of 30 (Rennie 2009). Muscle power, being the speed with which a muscle is used, is lost at an even faster rate of about 30 per cent per decade, which means that many older adults will find it difficult to rise from a chair unaided (Skelton *et al.* 1994). Another consequence of this decline is that 31 per cent of women over 70 are unable to walk a quarter of a mile (Skelton *et al.* 1994). In effect, this means that their world is restricted to about 200 metres radius from their home. This is a further consequence which has implications for social care costs (Abate *et al.* 2007).

The combined effect of reduced strength, inactivity and long spells of sedentary behaviour generates for many people an inactivity impairment, which constrains their quality of living and reduces their horizons. When one examines the evidence of functional decline and reduced levels of physical activity associated with ageing, it highlights the need to place a much higher priority on the importance of promoting regular physical activity for all older people. This impoverished situation is preventable, so what is standing in the way of people doing more physical activity? It is clear that very many older adults are not physically literate. They are not motivated to take part in any form of physical activity, with the consequences mentioned above.

Understanding why people do not exercise enough

There have been a considerable number of research reports which have explored people's motivation and the determinants of inactivity patterns of those who are unwilling or unable to participate regularly in physical activity. There is a wealth of information within this research but there may well be very basic issues that need to be addressed first. In this section, three specific critical issues that dominate the British Heart Foundation National Centre's (BHFNC) work with older adults will be considered.

The first issue is that engaging in purposeful physical pursuits, such as walking, gardening or involvement in some form of physical activity, is a low priority in people's lives (HSE 2008). This situation needs to be addressed. For most adults 30 minutes of physical activity represents only 2 per cent of their day, yet the majority of adults will spend at least 16 per cent of their day sitting in front of a television or computer screen. 'Not having enough time' is not an adequate explanation; it is simply that adults do not recognise daily physical activity as a priority in their lives. This is reinforced when one examines how often people are physically active at weekends. Compared with weekdays adults are less active at weekends when, theoretically, they have more time.

The second issue is the lack of understanding where almost the whole population has some difficulty with the public health message. It is quite clear from discussions with many adults that they have difficulty understanding the physical activity message and what they need to do. There is some evidence that only 3 per cent of men and 7 per cent of women in the 55 to 64 age range (DoH 2009a) know what the current physical activity recommendations are. Focus groups with older adults aged 55 to 65 (BHF 2008a) report very little understanding of what is entailed in 30 minutes of moderate activity on five or more days a week. The media compound the problem by citing different research projects that appear to contradict each other. As a result, the picture for many adults is confusing.

In fact this second issue is further compounded by the diversity of the population called 'older' adults. This is particularly important because the older adult could be a very active 55-year-old woman, a 68-year-old man exercising daily with two medical conditions, a person who has never exercised for 40 years, an active 95-year-old woman living independently or a very frail 80-year-old man. The range is extensive. Guidelines need to take account of the diversity of older adults' populations. They need to avoid a 'catch-all' policy. Yet, in the UK there is very little guidance to provide support in the promotion of more purposeful physical pursuits for older adults. In response to this problem the BHFNC launched a consultation document together with a series of regional seminars where this issue was explored in greater depth in order to understand the nature of the problem. This new guidance document (BHF 2009) was an attempt to provide more comprehensive and informed advice to all those working with older adults.

A third issue was identified in the BHFNC Older People media campaign (30 a day 2008b). A report was commissioned by the BHF to explore attitudes. One disturbing point that emerged was that 62 per cent of the sample reported that they would not be motivated to exercise even if their life depended on it (BHF 2007). This illustrates what a complex problem we are dealing with in trying to convince people that regular physical activity has value. For older adults they often cite their age and the presence of some limiting medical conditions together with a sense of fatalism as reasons why they cannot undertake sufficient exercise on a daily basis (Sport England 2006b).

When one considers these problems, it would seem that we have failed to demonstrate that physical activity or indeed physical literacy can be a powerful force in promoting well-being, enabling people to flourish and enrich their lives. For many researchers, the solution lies in social marketing (French 2008), identifying key messages, exploring the needs, interests and aspirations of segmented groups and using this information appropriately, with specific targeted populations. Of course, this can be a valuable tool but in terms of physical literacy we need first of all to explore the image that we present of purposeful physical pursuits.

The promotion of physical activity

There is a powerful case for promoting the idea that more people should be more active more often (DoH 2004b). More recently 'Be Active Be Healthy: a plan for getting the nation moving' (DoH 2009a), has been compiled and provides evidence to demonstrate the effective role physical activity can play in the treatment of specific medical conditions, and identifies the major economic benefits of getting the nation more active. In an analysis of documents that promote physical activity and health, it is usual to associate physical activity with two roles: first, therapy and treatment of specific medical conditions, and second, in terms of preventing ill-health and reducing the risks of acquiring specific conditions. Physical activity is very often seen as an instrumental tool to support therapeutic or treatment programmes. Of course, this is valuable and primary care teams need to ensure that effective programmes are in place. However, this approach alone is inadequate. Thus, this leads decision-makers to highlight the second role of a preventive agenda for physical activity.

For example, in terms of older adults the prevention agenda is advocated on the grounds that it will:

- reduce the risk for specific medical conditions
- delay functional decline
- delay dependency
- prevent the complications of immobility.

Thus, the justification for the promotion of regular physical activity in strategy documents highlights the economic cost of inactivity and the need for a prevention action plan. However, there is a major problem with the prevention agenda because it tends to be associated with a negative message: 'If you don't exercise regularly you put yourself at risk from acquiring a number of medical conditions which could reduce your life expectancy, constrain your ability to maintain your health at an optimal level and influence your well-being.' People are warned of the dangers of ill-health caused by lifestyle factors that can be avoided. Thus, the message is that taking part in more physical activity will reduce the risk of developing specific conditions and save the health service considerable sums of money.

However, it is quite clear that this negative approach has failed because large numbers of people have not been convinced that they should become more active. The way that the prevention agenda is presented may be at fault because it is clearly more important to halt or delay the development of specific conditions than wait until people have developed a condition. If a positive message and a different image of purposeful physical pursuits were to be promoted, it could be possible to address the prevention agenda without the association with negative messages. There is a need for a more positive message that reaches individual people, engages their interest and stimulates action.

A positive perspective for purposeful physical pursuits and physical literacy

In a series of 34 focus groups (Sport England 2007) with sedentary adults, who had joined a workplace programme to encourage people to become more physically active in a wide variety of activities and maintained their commitment over a whole year, most of the participants said that the main reason for staying with the programme was 'I have more energy now'. This is an important point because they associated their new vitality and energy with being active on a regular basis. This is a powerful argument for exploring how we can encourage people to make a commitment to being active and represents an important start for a new message.

This research provides us with a starting point to address a positive perspective for the promotion of purposeful physical pursuits. This term is preferred to physical activity as it has wider connotations and avoids the specific association with types of 'sports' activities. Purposeful physical pursuits include walking, cycling, gardening and housework. We need to use the idea that purposeful physical pursuits can energise lives, enabling people to feel that they have more vitality and dynamism.

As part of the development of the Moving More Often programme (BHF 2008c) adults' feelings were taken into account. In discussions with older adults who were asked 'what would make life better?' the following three points were highlighted. They would like to:

- talk with someone regularly
- get out more
- do something.

It is interesting that these responses are similar to studies with young people where they identify that they would like to:

- talk with friends
- have places to go
- have something to do.

The results of this study formed the basis for action by community nurses who identified people, usually women, living independently but who rarely left their house or flat and experienced isolation. The experiences of Phyllis (Case study 10.1) are an example of the benefits of purposeful physical pursuits.

Case study 10.1 Phyllis

Phyllis lived alone and rarely ventured outside her home. She was however persuaded to go out and walk to the local post office and shops where she could talk with other people. These walks were extended on a more regular basis and Phyllis became more confident of walking longer distances. She was persuaded to meet with people who went on a weekly walk from a leisure centre. This set in motion a series of events. Phyllis started to walk more often and meet with her friends and, after a period of time she felt more confident, much fitter and was able to walk for longer periods.

At the leisure centre she noted that people, younger than her, played a variety of games such as badminton, table tennis and tennis which she had never played. She persuaded a friend to go with her and they asked for help to try these games. Friendly members of staff were only too happy to help and soon Phyllis was able to enjoy playing and experiencing the thrill of learning new skills. Her whole world changed. She had friends to do things with and she had the capacity to get out and undertake challenging activities in a social context. For Phyllis, getting out and starting to walk with friends was the beginning of a more enriched life. In other words, walking, talking with friends and playing games widened her perspectives, enabled her to extend her capabilities and improved the quality of living immeasurably.

Phyllis learned to love being active in her eighties. In fact it would appear that she became physically literate, that is, motivated to take part in activity. The beneficial outcomes are clear to see. The idea of enriching lives is exactly the same for Phyllis as it is with young mothers, children in early years, young adults leaving school, or middle-aged men and women. This example illustrates a second feature of a positive message to promote purposeful physical pursuits – enriching lives. This idea of enriching lives by engagement in purposeful physical pursuits supported by a social context represents a powerful reason for introducing a whole range of physical activities to both young and old.

However, we need to emphasise that enriching lives is about widening perspectives, extending horizons of what individuals are capable of doing, acquiring confidence, achieving a sense of success and feeling good about what has been achieved. In the above example it was also the social context that reinforced the commitment to being active, as this can extend an individual's social contacts and build new social networks. In this more positive perspective on the value of purposeful physical pursuits, the role of physical activity may be seen as building a well-being resource and enabling people to flourish in two ways. It is suggested that purposeful physical pursuits can:

- energise lives
- enrich lives.

If this approach works and we can persuade more people to be more active more of the time and recognise that regular, purposeful physical pursuits are important for their well-being, the health benefits of this commitment will naturally accrue. This will enable us to tackle the prevention agenda at the same time with no extra resources or cost. These points are important because a more positive and personal message can present purposeful physical pursuits in a different light since the activity levels of older adults are exceptionally low. Instead of highlighting just the role that regular physical activity can play in reducing the risks of particular medical conditions, we need to focus on the central role that physical activity can play in living life to the full whatever your age. In addition, we can help the general public to understand that even people with medical conditions can exercise safely, and this will help in the management of those medical conditions amenable to exercise and enable people to experience the health benefits of activity.

This position leads to the role of purposeful physical pursuits in physical literacy. The recognition and promotion of the value of physical literacy as a lifespan issue operating from an early age through to the third age has much to offer. In other words, physical literacy has relevance to the whole lifecourse where the challenges of promoting purposeful physical pursuits with very young children are similar to those of working with older adults.

Physical literacy can provide an overarching concept that goes beyond the simple provision of opportunities for being active. In the next section this position will be developed in greater depth.

Physical literacy

Whitehead has worked to propound the value of physical literacy over a number of years. She has provided a conceptual framework of the meaning of physical literacy and outlined a number of convincing arguments (Whitehead 2006, 2007a) for the promotion of this capability. The framework that she outlines should be considered as a starting point for informing our thinking of how physical literacy can be transformed into a practical tool. In the spirit of this approach a number of developments to her framework may be suggested to illustrate how the concept can be applied to the challenge of promoting physical activity with older adults. As set out in Chapter 2, Whitehead outlines the *short* definition of physical literacy in the following terms: As appropriate to each individual's endowment, physical literacy may be described as 'the motivation, confidence, physical competence, knowledge and understanding to maintain physical activity throughout the lifecourse'.

Further detail in Chapter 2 includes the suggestions that:

> Physical literacy may be described as a disposition characterised by the motivation and confidence to capitalise on innate movement potential to make a significant contribution to the quality of life.
>
> In addition, physically literate individuals will have the ability to identify and articulate the essential qualities that influence the effectiveness of their own movement performance, and have an understanding of the principles of embodied health, with respect to basic aspects such as exercise, sleep and nutrition.

Whitehead goes on to articulate a number of other characteristics; however, the two cited above have been highlighted as they are important aspects in respect of the older adult population. It could be helpful to develop on from these baseline descriptions to identify a number of additional factors, possibly implicit in Whitehead's concept of physical literacy, that are particularly pertinent. With particular reference to the older adult population, but relevant to all, the following could be seen to fill out and further enrich the description of a physically literate individual. An individual who is physically literate displays:

- a love of being physically active;
- the physical competence, motivation, confidence and understanding to:
  - recognise the value of a physically active lifestyle to energise life and enrich the quality of living;

- engage in a range of physical activities on a regular basis because of the satisfactions inherent in their pursuit;
- appreciate their contribution to personal well-being and seek to engage regularly in purposeful physical activities;

- the maintenance of this commitment at an individually appropriate level throughout the lifecourse;
- a recognition of the need for a personal responsibility to enhance well-being and contribute to the well-being of others.

These characteristics provide further details that inform the development of physical literacy for and in individual lives. However, the concept of physical literacy and its associated characteristics will have no value unless they can be applied to and influence common practice. Promoting physical literacy needs to be seen as a guide to practice, a guide that enables practitioners to acquire an intelligent and informed perspective on the potential of purposeful physical activity in people's lives.

This process entails recognition of a role in lifelong education to promote physical activity and thus physical literacy. In this instance, people, whether they are young or old, need to learn how they can come to value physical literacy. Second, this educational role is associated with a pedagogy – how do we engage with people? This process of engagement is about connecting with people, whether young or old, to facilitate the growth of understanding in appreciating and valuing an engagement in a variety of purposeful physical activities, so that they can acquire a commitment that lasts a lifetime. It is this process that needs to be identified and developed further, together with an idea of what kinds of activities stimulate engagement and commitment.

Physical literacy and lifelong education

The programmes that are devised to develop physical literacy are advised to use purposeful physical activities because they can enhance lives and improve the quality of living. These activities have the power to enrich and transform lives, become an absorbing interest that rewards and fulfils, and also provide avenues for the enhancement of human capacities and qualities. The task of a facilitator, be they teacher, pedagogue, mentor, coach, personal trainer, practitioner and parent, is to help people acquire a commitment to being active informed by the satisfactions aroused by the pursuit of specific purposeful physical activities whether this is dance, a game or simply walking in the countryside. These satisfactions can generate a feeling of success and enjoyment shared with friends, and can lead to a love of being active. These can be the beginnings of developing physical literacy, with the attendant commitment that can enhance well-being, improve health and enable individuals to flourish as persons.

We need to recognise this important role of stimulating new interests and widening people's perspectives about the richness and potential of the vast range of purposeful pursuits available. People need to learn how to engage in purposeful pursuits, to make choices and select activities that can contribute to the enrichment of their lives and add immensely to the quality of daily living. However, people need to go beyond engagement, they need also to learn how to appreciate, value and learn from their engagement. In this way they are making choices about what they can do with their lives that lead to an informed and intelligent use of their time and effort. The central features of physical literacy need to be made accessible to all, from the very young who have unformed and uninformed minds and whose ability to evaluate life plans and make choices about what to do with their lives is not yet developed, through to those of an older age. It is therefore important for a lifelong educational strategy to be developed for promoting purposeful physical pursuits and, through this, physical literacy. The importance of physical literacy in society and individual communities cannot be overlooked.

If we are to help people to learn how to lead full and valuable lives by engaging in purposeful pursuits, what does this entail? People need to learn how to value pursuits in a rich and fundamental way by coming to care about them. The way we engage in pursuits, understanding what they entail, appreciating the satisfactions that can be generated and learning how to make informed choices can lead to an understanding of how we can spend our time productively. In promoting physical literacy we are striving to help people get on the inside of different physical pursuits so that they learn to appreciate what they can offer, value their commitment and learn to care about their participation. This is an important role because it opens up new perspectives that can add quality and meaning to one's life. It is not good enough simply to provide people with opportunities to engage in purposeful physical pursuits. We need practitioners with the professional and educational skills to engage with people and help them to learn to love being active and care about their involvement. They need the skills to cultivate, nurture and help people to cherish their sense of vitality, energy and well-being, and avoid squandering the very essence of living.

There is one additional issue that needs to be considered in this context. If we are able to help people to get on the inside of purposeful pursuits and enjoy the satisfactions inherent therein and learn to develop a commitment, they need to recognise the need for personal responsibility. A person's well-being can only be promoted if they accept that it is in their own hands to do all they can to enhance their life; no one else can do this. It is therefore essential that individuals acknowledge that they are responsible for their own life choices.

In the context of physical literacy, when we speak of an 'educational role' it can suggest that we are dealing with only young people. However, in working to promote physical literacy, cradle to grave, this 'education' needs to be a lifelong experience. Thus, all those working with others, namely personal trainers, mentors, leisure professionals, movement and exercise tutors, need to adopt the same professional skills required by teachers. We have been singularly unsuccessful in demonstrating the value of purposeful physical pursuits to large numbers of people. In the same way that teachers and practitioners work with young people, we are striving to open the minds and hearts of older adults to the satisfactions that can be generated from purposeful physical pursuits. This theoretical position needs to be supported by 'educational practices' that engage people.

Physical literacy and a pedagogy of engagement

What does a pedagogy of engagement entail? We tend to use the term pedagogy in a broad and loose way as the science and principles of teaching but it is rare for teachers to develop this further and articulate its relevance for enhancing their practice. Recently, the idea of pedagogy has been revived and there is now considerable academic interest in educational circles (DfES 2004). Nevertheless, this work has not touched on the teaching of physical activities, even though there is some interest in developing strategies for teaching and learning. Pedagogy needs to be seen in terms of the art and science of engaging with students to stimulate productive learning. This stipulative statement focuses on engagement with learners. What does this engagement entail? A framework for good practice in which it was recommended that teachers adopt strategies to help young people acquire positive interpersonal relationships was outlined by Almond (1997). These proposals subsequently informed work with teachers who wanted to improve their practice. While these were written with school-age students in mind they are equally pertinent to work with older adults.

One scenario captures this work neatly and illustrates that a pedagogy of engagement can emerge. After an OFSTED inspection a number of school staff who were seen as failing teachers in need of help were paired with experienced and successful colleagues. In failing to raise standards it was felt that a breakdown in communications with young people and an inability to create a productive working environment was the source of the problem. The experienced teachers began to explore the perceived problem and came up with a list of skills that would help their colleagues to be more successful. The following items were seen as crucial skills that could be practised and refined. There was a need to:

- reach out to all students;
- establish a connection with individual students that enables learning to take place;
- engage with students productively, with enthusiasm and empathy;
- draw students out with challenges that excite, engage their interest and allow them to develop with confidence;
- stretch students' abilities, interests and love of learning.

This became the focus for the mentoring work with less successful teachers. Over a number of weeks the teachers practised these skills, refined what worked well and reflected on how they could develop ideas that would capture the imagination of their students. In this process they learned confidence, a recognition of what teaching could be like and a greater understanding of their students.

The skills outlined above represent a set of core competences, not simply technical skills because the teachers needed to apply them in context with an understanding of the students with whom they were working. Thus, technical competences need appropriate practice, critical reflection, refinement and a recognition that they are employed in the interests of promoting a love of learning. We need to explore further the relationship between the art and science of engagement. A pedagogy of engagement is central to the art of promotion whether it is academic learning or learning to love being active with young people or older adults.

While the brief discussion of a pedagogy of engagement above referred to teachers in school, the skills of engagement are relevant for a much wider range of professionals. Practitioners in early years settings, mentors, personal trainers, health trainers, lifestyle coaches, social care workers, sport coaches and adults working with older adults need to be aware of these practical recommendations and appreciate their importance in the promotion of physical literacy. Chapter 13 looks at the range of significant others involved in nurturing physical literacy, and Chapter 14 discusses learning and teaching approaches to foster physical literacy.

Promoting purposeful physical pursuits with older adults

How can these ideas inform the practice of people working with older adults? The British Heart Foundation National Centre developed a range of resources and training programmes to enable professionals to capture the imagination of older adults and stimulate more purposeful physical pursuits, with the goal of helping older adults to energise and enrich their lives. At the same time, there was a recognition that there is an educational role and a need to engage productively with older adults underpinning all aspects of the training.

'Someone Like Me' (Laventure *et al.* 2008) is a peer mentoring resource to encourage older adults to help other older adults to become more interested in being active and provide a support to those who find it difficult to maintain a commitment. Older adults who attend the training courses have the opportunity to learn skills of engaging with their colleagues and learn how to promote more activity more of the time. In this context the mentors are adopting an educational role and using pedagogy to reach out to people. In the same way health trainers, lifestyle consultants, life coaches and other forms of mentors can benefit from a recognition of their educational and pedagogical roles. A programme entitled 'Moving More

Often' has also been developed to enable care homes to provide purposeful physical pursuits to encourage residents to be more active. A number of different modules such as Games People Play, Walk with Me, Out and About, Just Me, Dance with Me, Gardening, Tai Chi and Wii were developed so that staff could implement them in individual care homes according to preference and availability. These initiatives have raised participation rates considerably because they have energised residents' lives and enabled them to enrich their living.

In Wales and Yorkshire two areas have gone beyond this programme and introduced the idea of a care homes' Olympic festival which they called an Olympiage. In an Olympiage men and women from different care homes take part in a festival where residents are involved in a range of purposeful physical pursuits. The celebration of an Olympiage achieved all its aspirations. It created a new 'can do' spirit among residents, stimulated more social networks and gave people a range of challenges. In addition, it gave residents something to look forward to and persuaded the staff in care homes to rethink the value of purposeful physical pursuits. The festivals generated considerable interest, including media attention, and attracted acclaim from different sources when the enjoyment, smiles and physical abilities of the participants were clear to see. Further development of this initiative would dispel the image of care homes as places where residents were predominantly inactive. It would allow residents to take part in a range of purposeful physical pursuits and to be involved in preparing for an outing. It would provide opportunities for richer social contact and enable residents to associate themselves with the Olympics. If this idea were to spread widely it would be possible to see a real legacy from the 2012 Olympics. Each town and city in the UK could promote a Care Homes Olympiage prior to the Olympic Games. This would be a real achievement and provide a significant image of just what older adults are capable of. It would indeed send out a very powerful media message. However, there is a long way to go before we can encourage all care homes to see physical activity as a way of enriching and energising lives.

Following the BHFNC media campaign of 30 a day, last year, a comprehensive document on guidelines for promoting purposeful physical pursuits with older adults was developed. In this new resource (BHF 2009) guidelines have been developed for professionals working with older adults on how they can develop programmes and use evidence-based interventions with older adults. The resources include recommendations about what kinds of purposeful physical pursuits would be appropriate and how physical activity can be very effective in promoting well-being and enriching lives.

Conclusion

This chapter has attempted to do four things:

- extend the notion of physical literacy to address particular needs in the older adult population;
- propose the use of the term purposeful physical pursuits;
- identify an educational role and a pedagogy of engagement that under-pins a commitment to promote physical literacy;
- endorse the view that the promotion of physical literacy is relevant to all age groups and should be seen as a lifespan concern.

The introduction of the term purposeful physical pursuits in preference to the rather narrow concept of physical activity is particularly important in having much richer connotations. The term enables one to associate activity with the need for an educational and pedagogical stance to physical literacy. This stance enables physical literacy to be seen in a practical context that may be applied in everyday practice.

As a lifespan issue, purposeful physical pursuits lie at the heart of being physically literate. Whether one works in early years settings or with older adults, there is a need to encourage everyone to love being active. The low levels of physical activity in the adult population, particularly those beyond the age of 65, indicate that we have failed to generate this love. An understanding of physical literacy with its educational and pedagogical implications provides the opportunity to challenge traditional practice and highlight a powerful tool for enhancing the lives of everyone.

Recommended reading

Liu, C.J. and Latham, N.K. (2009) Progressive resistance strength training for improving physical function in older adults. *Cochrane Database of Systematic Reviews* 3.

Ratey, J.J. and Hagerman, E. (2008) *SPARK: The Revolutionary New Science of Exercise and the Brain*. Little, Brown & Company, New York.

11 Physical literacy and individuals with a disability

Philip Vickerman and Karen DePauw

Introduction

This chapter considers the promotion of physical literacy in individuals with a disability, throughout their lifecourse. It explores the importance of physical literacy to these individuals while examining how it can be achieved within their unique environmental settings. International statements on the entitlement of those with a disability are included, as are definitions of disability and types of barriers these individuals may meet. A key focus of the chapter will be to identify best practice strategies that aim to foster the confidence, self-esteem and motivation of these individuals in physical activity contexts, thus nurturing the development of their physical literacy. The benefits of being physically literate for those with a disability are addressed and exemplified by two case studies. Chapter 4 lays the ground for this discussion in arguing that physical literacy is a universal concept that all can achieve.

The entitlement of individuals with a disability to have opportunities to become physically literate

The increasing international emphasis on individuals' with disabilities entitlement to high-quality physical activity was crystallised through the Salamanca Statement (UNESCO 1994) which was signed by 92 governments and 25 international organisations. This established a set of beliefs and proclamations that every child has fundamental rights to education and identified core principles of providing children with the opportunity to learn, an education system designed to take account of diversity, access to regular child-centred education and the acceptance of inclusive orientation as a means of combating discrimination and building an inclusive society. The Salamanca Statement has, according to Farrell (2001), led to a plethora of legislation, policies and practices internationally (Booth *et al.* 1998) that focus upon children and adults with disabilities and their access to all aspects of society, including physical activity. Furthermore, the second World Summit on Physical Education (ICSSPE 2005) identified the distinctive focus of physical education on learning processes and teaching approaches while reaffirming its mission to support the inclusion of all children whatever their backgrounds and/or abilities.

Bee and Boyd (2006) suggest interpreting notions of disability and inclusion can be both complex and diverse. They encompass a range of issues related to the tensions and challenges of multidisciplinary approaches to supporting individuals becoming physically literate. According to Cameron and Murphy (2007), individuals with a disability lie upon a continuum in which there is often no clear-cut distinction between those who need additional intervention and those who do not. Conceptualising differences of disability on a continuum is therefore complicated and fraught with difficulties due to the many contrasting, and often opposing, views as to what counts as a disability (Dyson and Millward 2000).

The World Health Organisation (WHO) (2009) suggests that 'disability is a complex phenomenon, reflecting an interaction between features of a person's "body" and features of the society in which he or she lives'. The WHO goes on to explain that the term 'disability' is an umbrella term that encompasses impairments, activity limitations and participation restrictions. It suggests that 'impairment' is a problem in 'body' function or structure; whereas an 'activity limitation' refers to difficulties encountered by an individual in executing a task or action. Finally, the WHO refers to 'participation restriction' as a problem experienced by individuals in their involvement in life situations.

Burchardt (2004) suggests that 'social models of disability' create systemic barriers, negative attitudes and exclusion by society, intentionally or unintentionally, as the central factors in defining who is disabled or not. In addition, according to Reindal (2008), while some people have physical, sensory, intellectual or psychological variants which may cause individual functional limitation or impairments, these do not have to lead to disability. Thus as Reiser and Mason (1990) note, 'social models of disability' do not deny that some individual differences can lead to limitations but these are not the cause of individuals being excluded, rather it is societies' lack of flexibility to accommodate disabled people's needs that is the most significant limiting factor.

Inclusion in respect of promoting physical literacy must, therefore, focus on the unique needs of individuals with disabilities. Their personal potential must be a key feature throughout all aspects of any definitions and inter-pretations. This approach upholds the notion of the individual uniqueness of human beings and how they develop as embodied individuals (Whitehead 2007a). Thus, how individuals with disability evidence physical literacy will be specific to each of them, as will be the pace at which this capability develops (Wright and Sugden 1999). As was discussed in Chapter 3, every individual will be on their own physical literacy journey and progress should be judged in this context. This is in contrast to any attempts to measure certain aspects of physical literacy against standardised notions and expectations applied to non-disabled people.

Learning to move, moving to learn: developing confidence, motivation and self-esteem through physical activity

According to Sugden and Wright (1998), individuals with disabilities, like their non-disabled peers, need to experience physical activity, learning and development in a wide range of activities and environments. The rationale for supporting the development of disabled people's physical literacy is twofold: first, for individuals' own physical development, and second, as an essential component in promoting social, emotional, intellectual and cognitive development.

For children and adults with a disability, being physically literate enhances confidence, self-esteem, growth and development, fitness, and helps to teach them about their world. There is considerable awareness (Whitehead with Murdoch 2006; Vickerman 2007) of the contribution this capability can have on the physical, social, emotional and intellectual development of children with a disability. While all significant others have a role to play in this process, those leading physical education in schools have a key responsibility. Thus practitioners need to be aware of the effect that learning in a physical activity context can have on all-round development.

The relevance and importance of learning through physical activity cannot be overstated. In addressing this issue, Seaman and DePauw (1989) suggest becoming physically literate should be considered as a universal developmental process that is inclusive of (dis)ability. They argue that developmental approaches to physical literacy should employ a myriad of methods and techniques in predetermined and systematic ways to facilitate growth and development among individuals with 'performance disorders'. In adopting such an approach, disabled individuals may then achieve their maximum potential. Applying such methods allows for recognition of the individual as a unique embodied learner alongside identifying foundations for understanding causes of 'atypical' sequences of performance. Such personalised approaches to physical literacy are therefore defined as non-categorical and inclusive of the full diversity of disabled people's needs.

Another important point to consider in any discussion on ranges of disability is that according to Sugden and Wright (1998), not all will have difficulties in respect of physical competence. A child with emotional behavioural difficulties, for example, may excel in physical activity and a child with learning difficulties may be an excellent swimmer. Consequently, we should not assume that disability equals difficulty in physical competence and therefore development of physical literacy. In saying that, though, catering for individuals with disabilities generally does pose challenges for those encouraging or leading physical activity, and this is where having an open mind, high expectations and a willingness to adapt practices are critical to success.

Many disabilities can lead to a lack of confidence in individuals' management of their embodied dimension and this in turn can lead to difficulties in having positive experiences and being motivated to engage in physical activity (Weiss and Haber 1999; Wellard 2006). Therefore those responsible for physical activity throughout the lifecourse of these disabled individuals must ensure that the participants do not feel they are being limited in their physical activity experiences. It is also important that the promotion of physical literacy for individuals with a disability is not seen as of value purely in physical terms. Many activities, according to Sugden and Wright (1998), present additional opportunities to develop social skills that can lead to an independent life that is appropriate, pleasurable, creative and meets individual needs. An exciting activity programme can stimulate and motivate individuals who in turn are less likely to become frustrated or emotionally disturbed. Those with a disability should be given every opportunity and encouragement to use their embodied potential to the best of their ability.

The aims of involvement in physical activity for individuals with a disability are no different to those of any other person. They are entitled, through legislation in many countries, to a broad, balanced, progressive, differentiated and relevant programme of activities. Clearly, some will have greater difficulties than others in terms of active participation, but it is important that provision be made for their inclusion alongside their non-disabled peers. It is also important that, should it be necessary for an activity or equipment to be modified or substituted, the activity maintains its integrity and is in no way presented as a tokenistic gesture. Individuals with a disability by their very nature possess a wide range of personal and specific needs which have enormous complexity and diversity. To offer a comprehensive physical activity programme that caters for such diversity may present considerable challenges for practitioners. However, the movement competencies that are learned and experienced by disabled individuals will support them and carry them forward throughout their life (Kasser and Lytle 2005) while assisting them towards active and worthwhile roles within society.

Targeting barriers to participation to support the development of physical literacy

Barriers to individuals with disabilities becoming physically competent and thus physically literate have been subject to significant debate by authors such as Fredrickson and Cline (2002), Crawford *et al.* (2008), Nancy *et al.* (2008) and Reindal (2008). In acknowledgement of varying models of disability, Fredrickson and Cline (2002) suggest that a combination of individual differences, environmental demands and interactional analyses has contributed to differing perspectives on inclusion (Ballard 1997).

Individual models of inclusion consider barriers to becoming physically competent as being owned by the disabled individual. Thus, barriers to learning and development in physical activity are created by the diversity of an individual's disabilities (Reiser and Mason 1990) and the challenges these create. Exclusion or isolation, therefore, is not attributable to the environment, for example, in restrictions applied by those managing physical activity settings. Thus this model perceives a person's disability as the main barrier to becoming physically competent. Any lack of attempt by practitioners to accommodate these differences, by modifying existing structures and systems, is seen as secondary.

Burchardt (2004), in contrast, suggests environmental models in defining barriers to participation. These adopt situation, rather than person-centred, foci to supporting inclusive physical activity. Cole (2008) suggests that barriers to learning and access to high-quality physical activity can only be defined in terms of relationships between what an individual can do, and what practitioners do to enable success in any given environment. The limiting factor for any individual with a disability being able to develop physical competence rests, therefore, with practitioners adopting flexible approaches rather than expecting people to fit into existing structures. Barriers are considered to be created by lack of flexibility rather than any 'deficit' an individual may bring to the activity. According to this model those managing all forms of physical activity play a significant role in facilitating and/or constraining an individual's abilities to become physically competent and thus physically literate.

In drawing the similarities and differences of individual and environmental models of disability together, interactional models note the impossibility of separating the learning and physical competencies from the environment within which individuals live and function. Thus models of causation and location of barriers to physical literacy may be seen as a combination of complex interactions between the strengths and weaknesses of individuals, levels of support available, and the appropriateness of activities being provided. Thus neither environmental nor individual models exclusively describe the reality of inclusive practice. Rather, the central factor in supporting unique embodied experiences should be premised upon concern for high-quality experiences in physical activity made possible by appropriate support from knowledgeable practitioners sensitive to the wide range of individual needs (Rink and Hall 2008).

Strategies for promoting physical literacy in individuals with a disability

In order to maximise opportunities to support the development of physical literacy it is important that this is premised on addressing individual needs. Strategies to support physical literacy should be carefully planned, focused, and have a clear purpose of offering opportunities to experience success and satisfaction. According to Mouratidis *et al.* (2008), time should also be built into activities to allow for repetition and for raising the self-esteem of disabled individuals as embodied learners.

It is useful here to refer to guidance given in England by the Qualifications and Curriculum Authority (2007). The requirement here is for teachers to be sensitive to the specific needs of individuals with disabilities, while being non-judgemental and ready to recognise both effort and success. While the strategies set out below are designed to guide teachers, they are highly relevant to all those working in the movement field with individuals with a disability. The following principles of practice are recommended:

- *Setting suitable learning challenges*: Here physical education teachers and other practitioners in the field of physical activity should reflect the diversity of physical competence by developing different objectives based upon individual needs. A child who has a learning difficulty, for example, may find it difficult to verbalise a movement vocabulary but may be able to demonstrate competence through physical demonstration. In contrast, physically disabled children may struggle to demonstrate a particular movement pattern and/or activity but may be able to demonstrate verbally what aspects of physical competence mean for them (Vickerman 2007). In setting suitable learning challenges, teachers and other practitioners can ensure that individuals with disabilities are stretched and challenged to progress and achieve at a level and pace that meets their unique needs.

- *Responding to the diverse needs of pupils*: This leads to the second requirement for those promoting physical literacy. That is, to acknowledge difference and diversity, while embracing interactional models of disability, which seek to recognise the uniqueness of each individual and result in modifying activities as required (Reiser and Mason 1990; Fredrickson and Cline 2002). Thus, universal approaches are seldom appropriate to individuals with disabilities – rather acceptance and celebration of difference and diversity is central to fostering positive experiences of physical activity (Coates and Vickerman 2008).

- *Differentiating assessment and learning to meet individual needs of pupils*: If difference and diversity are to be embraced by teachers and other practitioners this will involve recognition that individuals with disabilities are all on a continuum of learning, and as such alternative methods of charting progress which maximise opportunities for all to demonstrate growing physical literacy should be established. If different learning challenges are offered to support the development of physical competence, then alternative methods of demonstrating competence should also be facilitated which reflect different stages of development. This has been referred to elsewhere in the book as the recording of individuals' progress on their personal journey to become, and to maintain, physical literacy.

The outcomes of adopting practices that follow from the principles set out above should include the rejection of any 'deficit' models of those with disabilities and the removal of any barriers to personal achievement. It is essential that all practitioners start from the premise that everyone can learn and develop if the right opportunities are provided for them.

Other writers support these principles. For example, Sugden and Keogh (1990) suggest that movement outcomes are determined by the interrelationship of three interacting variables of:

- the task to be performed
- the resources the child brings to the learning situation
- the context within which learning takes place.

In summary, three common factors recur in advice concerning catering for those with a disability. These are the need, first, to adapt both what is taught and the context in which the activity is taking place, second, to modify how guidance and support are given and finally to be sensitive to the needs of individuals with disabilities in respect of judging progress (Whitehead 2001; Fitzgerald 2005; Whitehead with Murdoch 2006).

It is pertinent here to comment on the role of physical education teachers in the promotion of physical literacy for those with a disability. These practitioners have a crucial part to play. Not only will they work with every child but they should be equipped, through their training, with sufficient knowledge and understanding to work effectively with pupils with a range of disabilities. This is backed up by the Association for Physical Education in the UK in their manifesto, which states: 'The aim of physical education is to develop physical competence so that all children are able to move efficiently, effectively and safely and understand what they are doing. The outcome, physical literacy, along with numeracy and literacy, is the essential basis for learners to access the whole range of competences and experiences' (afPE 2008). Physical education teachers are, therefore, charged with a particular responsibility to enact all the recommendations cited above.

The benefits of physical literacy

In working towards achieving the principles identified above, the following case studies (11.1 and 11.2) are offered to exemplify how individuals with a disability can access physical activity and in doing so become physically literate. The benefits of physical literacy are plain to see.

While it is the case that the fostering of physical literacy in school-age pupils is critical and should be a fundamental goal of physical education, physical literacy is an issue for all individuals at all stages of life. The implications of this are that there are many players in this enterprise beyond physical education teachers. In line with this, Aitchison (2003) argues that a significant goal is to ensure that all individuals with a disability, of whatever age, have the appropriate guidance and support to develop the motivation to engage in physical activity that is premised upon enhanced self-confidence and self-realisation. All individuals should experience success in respect of attaining and furthering their physical literacy. Indeed, the WHO (1997b) actively promotes health, well-being and physical activity among the full diversity of society. The WHO suggests that physical activity is an essential component of everyday life and appears to be the single, most effective means whereby individuals can influence health and functional well-being. Chapter 13 spells out the range of significant others who may be involved in fostering physical literacy, from the parent in the early years through to the carer working with elderly people.

Case study 11.1 Latisha

Latisha joined Beacon Hill School in September 2005, coming into year 7. She was a school refuser prior to joining the school. She was diagnosed with Autistic Spectrum Disorder, Tourettes Syndrome, Attention Deficit Hyperactivity Disorder and Separation Anxiety Disorder. When she started at Beacon Hill she had a very negative attitude towards the school, challenging staff and other pupils on a daily basis. Physical Education was an area where Latisha was able to excel and, due to the physical nature of the subject, she soon found that she was very capable of achieving success in a variety of activities and, when she was focused on tasks, she was less likely to show the symptoms of Tourettes. Through a variety of games, dance, gymnastics and athletic activities in PE Latisha slowly began to enjoy the success she was having and this started to have a positive impact on her confidence and self-esteem. As these improved, she was more willing to try new things and demonstrate her ability in front of her peers, something she refused to do when she first started. Through team sports such as basketball, she began to form more positive relationships with the other pupils. As a result, the social skills she developed in PE transferred into social times. Latisha is now in year 10 and currently undertaking the Sports Leaders UK Level 1 Award. She is a fantastic role model to her peers, showing responsibility and confidence when leading small groups. She works very well with younger pupils in the school, demonstrating patience and understanding. She takes pride in her appearance and has represented the school in different sporting activities, and also in London as a pupil voice of Building Schools for the Future.[1]

Case study 11.2 Thomas

Thomas joined Beacon Hill School in January 2008, coming into class 3. He was a very aggressive boy, diagnosed with ASD. When he first arrived, he completely changed the dynamics of the class with his challenging and violent behaviour, directed towards staff and pupils alike. During the first term of PE with Thomas, we were doing Sherborne Developmental Movement. In the beginning, he would fight to get away and would run off, refusing to interact with staff or other pupils. As we continued with the programme, we began to recognise that there were some interactions he liked. We gradually increased the time he had to 'rock' for and Thomas soon became confident and happy to sit and rock calmly with a member of staff. This was a very significant step in Thomas' progress and social interaction. From this, there was a significant improvement in Thomas' behaviour and how it was managed. He began to feel 'safe' with the adults, to develop trust and engage with them more positively. Thomas is now in class 4 and has had no violent incidents since he moved into this class. He is able to interact with other pupils at a socially acceptable level in PE, in the classroom and at social times. He is now a happy child who enjoys coming to school and is able to access other activities in PE such as gymnastics and team games. He is not only showing a significant improvement in his physical ability but his social skills, such as taking turns, listening and following instructions, have also improved. He is a pleasure to teach![2]

Movement development for individuals with a disability

Chapter 9 is devoted to movement development in the early years and addresses the importance of establishing an extensive movement vocabulary, mastering a range of movement patterns and developing movement capacities. As is pointed out in this chapter, physical competence is at the heart of physical literacy and thus is critical if this capability is to be fostered. While this is important for all young people, it is particularly crucial for those with a disability.

Although there are no distinctive stages in a child's movement development there are global phases the child passes through from birth to maturity. As a result, it is important to consider these phases from birth because many children with disabilities will show movement characteristics of children who are much younger. While age in years and months is not a totally accurate guide to development because of individual differences, it does offer some comparability to make judgements. This is particularly true of children with a disability whose developmental progress may vary dramatically and be delayed in comparison to those who are in 'standard' ranges – and this may continue to remain even in later childhood and through to adulthood. Indeed, it is likely that particular support and encouragement will be needed not only in childhood and adolescence but also after formal schooling is completed. It is surely the responsibility of any culture to continue to care for and make provision for those with a disability, throughout their lives. Chapter 10 considers ways in which the older adult population can be supported to attain or maintain physical literacy.

It is often the case that individuals with a disability are classified according to the severity of their particular conditions; however, while this can appear to be logical, it is not the most useful or productive manner in which to make progress. For example, there are some individuals with complex physical conditions who only require minimal adaptations, while others with fewer and less complex problems require significant intervention. Indeed, the need to adopt interactional approaches to disability by all those organising and leading physical activity is essential. Activities should be planned around individuals, rather than expecting them to fit into pre-existing environmental contexts. Physical literacy will only be developed if those with a disability have positive experiences in physical activity.

Sugden and Keogh (1990) and Sugden and Henderson (1994) cover a range of developmental phases and stages with particular reference to individuals with a disability. Both are valuable texts to study in more detail.[3]

Conclusion

Learning to move with confidence is central to individuals with a disability becoming physically literate. Success is not acquired naturally, nor is it genetic, and as such is dependent upon all practitioners developing effective strategies to create access and realise entitlement to individuals becoming physically competent. Some individuals with a disability will enjoy physical activity much more than others and as such will quickly develop their physical literacy where the right opportunities are provided. In contrast, some may have negative experiences of attempts to develop this capability and this can lead to a lack of motivation, confidence and self-esteem.

This chapter, building from arguments presented in Part I, has endorsed that everyone, regardless of their (dis)ability, can attain physical literacy. How this is then developed from an individual's unique embodied experience will be determined by several internal and external factors. These include an individual's attitude, self-confidence and motivation, alongside practitioners' commitment to develop environments that are conducive to learning. The chapter has also noted that physical activities for disabled individuals like their non-disabled peers are made up of essential movement patterns and movement capacities. These areas of movement competence underpin effective involvement in more structured forms pf physical activity. It is the case therefore that an inability to execute basic movement competences effectively can lead to low self-perception, feelings of frustration and disengagement.

The issue of supporting individuals with a disability in becoming physically literate can therefore be complex. In order to achieve this goal it is essential to make best use of the full range of individuals' unique embodied capacities in their interaction with the world. It may also be the case that focusing on different or restricted clusters of physical competencies evident in the disabled individual may make the best use of movement potential. However, practitioners will always have to balance the tensions between creating individualised programmes (Norwich 2002) to promote physical competence and the need to facilitate sessions that are inclusive to all. In meeting this goal, consideration of the following four factors is central to the success of the enterprise:

- *The holistic nature of a person*: At all times the individual must be seen as a unique whole. Celebrating difference and diversity and seeking maximum opportunities to develop and demonstrate physical literacy in as many ways as possible is paramount.
- *The importance of our relationship to the environment in which we live*: Effective interaction with the environment can make or break success in physical literacy. In this respect practitioners leading physical activity have a key responsibility in creating environments in which all can learn, thrive and progress.
- *The role of movement in wider development*: This factor serves to remind practitioners that physical literacy is not solely focused on enhancing physical competence but can make a significant contribution to the enhancement of other aspects of the person, such as language development, interaction with others and the ability to understand movement and how their embodiment functions in respect of health and well-being (Gallagher 2005).
- *The role of movement in developing a sense of self*: It should never be forgotten that an individual's embodiment is integral to their personhood. As is also discussed fully in Chapter 7, attitudes towards embodiment influence global self-esteem and self-confidence, and contribute to the development of a secure sense of self. This reinforces the role which becoming physically literate can have in supporting individuals with a disability in coming to understand themselves and their relationship to the world.

In summary, Whitehead (2007a) suggests that the potential of individuals with a disability to realise physical literacy underpins the assertion that all can acquire this capability, albeit in line with their individual endowment. All expressions of this capability will be particular to the individual. All expressions will widen opportunities and enhance life throughout the lifecourse. Those with physical disabilities should not be denied the opportunity to become physically literate. This chapter challenges all those with responsibilities for these individuals to make this a reality.

Recommended reading

Coates, J. and Vickerman, P. (2008) Let the children have their say: children with special educational needs experiences of physical education – a review. *Support for Learning*, 23, 4: 168–175.

This journal article will be useful in appreciating how disabled children can be given opportunities to have a 'voice' and be consulted on their experiences, views and opinions of physical activity. The article provides a comprehensive overview of strategies that have been used to empower disabled children to speak up and will be useful in assisting you with strategies for consultation.

Cole, R. (2008) *Educating Everybody's Children: Diverse Strategies for Diverse Learners, Association for Supervision and Curriculum Development.* Google Books. Online. Available http: <http://www.books.google.co.uk/books?id=ixm W-porsOAC> (accessed 22 August 2009).

This text provides a comprehensive overview of the diversity of children's needs. The book addresses a range of strategies that can be used to assist with maximising learning potential and will be of use to all those supporting learning and development of young people.

Fitzgerald, H. (2005) Still feeling like a spare piece of luggage? Embodied experiences of (dis)ability in physical education and school physical activity. *Physical Education and Physical Activity Pedagogy*, 10, 1: 41–59.

This journal article provides a unique insight into the experiences of disabled people in relation to their engagement with physical activity.

12 Physical literacy and issues of diversity

Philip Vickerman and Karen DePauw

Introduction

This chapter discusses issues concerned with promoting physical literacy in the context of diversity. It sets out to examine how issues of diversity relate to the opportunities for, and limitations of, individuals becoming physically literate. It will define the nature of diversity and why some individuals and groups may experience less supportive contexts than others. The chapter will also examine strategies to promote physical literacy among these diverse groups (Pecek *et al.* 2008) and what significant others in physical activity settings should do to facilitate inclusive physical activity. International statements on entitlement are included as are issues around equality of opportunity. Three areas of discussion will be addressed. These are concerned with physical literacy in relation to gender, to sexual orientation, and to religion, race and culture.

Context

The World Education Forum (2000) set out at the dawn of the twenty-first century to ensure that inclusive approaches to learning and teaching were adopted, and which accommodate the full diversity of all members of society. Indeed, the United Nations (UN) (2008) promotion of 'Education for All' set out to increase participation and learning for children who were perceived to be vulnerable to marginalisation or barriers to learning. The aim of creating inclusive approaches to learning, including becoming physically literate, should, according to Booth *et al.* (2000), be premised upon seeking to eliminate social exclusion and promote diversity of opportunity with a particular focus on issues of race, social class, ethnicity, religion and gender. Vickerman *et al.* (2003) propose that equality of opportunity in all physical activity settings including physical education should therefore focus upon celebration of difference and diversity (Cole 2008) that is matched by a commitment to treat people differently but fairly according to their individual needs. Differences should be seen as strengths not barriers or limitations to participation in physical activity. In this context, everyone should have the opportunity or indeed the right to become physically literate, expressed in ways that reflect and support their individual diversity.

Creating a precise definition of inclusion and diversity can be problematic due to the complexity of those to whom it refers. Booth and colleagues (2000: 12) suggest that within an educational context, for example,

> inclusion is a set of never ending processes. It involves the specification of the direction of change. It is relevant to any school however inclusive or exclusive its current cultures, policies and practices. . . . It requires schools to engage in a critical examination of what can be done to increase the learning and participation of the diversity of students within the school locality.

In contrast, Ballard (1997: 244) suggests that inclusion and diversity should be 'non-discriminatory in terms of disability, culture, gender or other aspects of students or staff that are assigned significance by a society'. He goes on the say that it involves all members of society with no exceptions and irrespective of their intellectual, physical, sensory or other differences. 'As such inclusion emphasises diversity over assimilation, striving to avoid the colonisation of minority experiences by dominant modes of thought and action' (Ballard 1997: 244). It is not surprising in this complex situation that in facilitating diversity in promoting physical literacy there are no easy strategies that address every individual's needs (Artilies 1998). Rather, what is required in respect of all those who play a part in fostering physical literacy throughout the lifecourse is a commitment to respond to individual diversity proactively, to have high expectations, and to be ready to modify and adapt learning, teaching and assessment practices as necessary.

In attempting to draw this variety of issues together with regard to physical literacy, it is necessary to examine what the specific issues are that may limit participation in physical activity. As part of this analysis, an examination of international perspectives on equality and diversity (Dyson and Millward 2000) will be considered in an attempt to identify and remove potential barriers to access and engagement in physical activity.

Equality of opportunity in physical literacy

According to Whitehead (2007a), there is a strong argument that everyone should have the opportunity to become physically literate. As the foundations of physical literacy are significantly and uniquely rooted in participation in physical activity, there should be equality of opportunity for individuals to become involved in physical activity, regardless of their individual needs. These opportunities should be premised upon fairness, while recognising any inequalities, and subsequently taking steps to address these differences (Bailey 2005). Entitlement and accessibility to experiences that establish and promote physical competence should therefore seek to change the culture and structure of any physical activity, to ensure this is barrier free to all members of society, whatever their age, gender, race, ethnicity, sexuality or socio-economic status.

In promoting this view the UN Resolution 56/75, instigated in 2002, reinforced the message of equality and diversity in physical activity through its Olympic movement goals. These set out to build a peaceful and better world through physical activity which is practised without discrimination of any kind and in the Olympic spirit which requires mutual understanding, friendship, solidarity and fair play. The UN (2008) ideals and commitments to diversity are not something new. Indeed, the European Physical Activity for All Charter (European Union (EU) 1992) which was revised in 2001 set out to provide a common framework to which all European countries can put their name. Alongside this, the EU Code of Physical Activity Ethics (1992) also works towards fair play as an essential element of all physical activities. In addition, as part of the EU Physical Activity Charter (EU 1992), governments have committed themselves to provide their citizens with opportunities to practise physical activity under well-defined conditions in which participation is accessible to everybody; is healthy and safe; fair and tolerant; builds on high ethical values; and is capable of fostering personal self-fulfilment at all levels.

Identification of the development of self-fulfilment is in line with suggestions that physical literacy can foster self-confidence and can enrich life. As suggested in Chapter 4, as human beings all individuals exhibit the potential to be physically literate, albeit the manner in which this is expressed may be different and/or particular to each individual depending on physical potential, self-identity and the cultural context. A physically literate individual, irrespective of diversity, will have a well-established sense of 'self' in relation to the world. This will be founded on the development of confident physical competence and fluent interaction with the environment, with the attendant development of self-esteem. Diversity should not stand in the way of this potential. All those who play a part in promoting physical activity need to display a sensitivity to the differences of those individuals with whom they are working. Underpinning this will be the need to understand the world from the standpoint of others, being alert to the realities which characterise differences in individuals' worlds.

Physical literacy and its relationship to specific groups

In societies across the world we are fortunate to have diverse populations (Wellard 2006) which are made up of a multiplicity of groups and individuals. In the twenty-first century, and as part of the modern world, diversity should be considered as a strength and something that should be celebrated. Supporting such diversity in the context of physical activity involves embracing the backgrounds and experiences of individuals and the potential they all have to become physically literate. It is a sad fact, however, that many people who take part in physical activity, as well as in other activities, are discriminated against, bullied, marginalised or even harassed on the basis of their individual diversity. As far back as 1948 the UN Declaration on Human Rights established fundamental recognition of individuals and groups to certain freedoms of expression. This was supplemented in a European context via The Council of Europe Convention on Human Rights which was established in 1950, and has since set out several protocols in relation to supporting diverse groups and individuals. The Convention notes that all human beings are born free and are entitled to equality of respect in relation to dignity and rights. Since the UN and Council of Europe Human Rights Charters, several additions and amendments have been made that reflect the shifting acceptance of societies to equality of opportunity irrespective of what that difference may be. However, in every one of the 192 member states signing up to the UN Human Rights Charter there are exclusions based on countries' individual perceptions and laws, some of which would seem to challenge contemporary views of equality.

In attempting to draw together the international Charters on Human Rights and the range of diversity of individuals and groups to which it refers, this chapter will now turn to an examination of the situation of specific individuals in the context of physical activity and hence the opportunity to become physically literate. The intention of the following sections is to raise awareness of the potential issues and barriers that may limit participation and engagement in physical activity. In doing so, it is not the intention to provide simple solutions to what are by their very nature complex issues. Rather, this section sets out to identify general principles that significant others who provide opportunities for physical activity can apply with respect to all individuals, while at the same time acknowledging and celebrating diversity.

Physical literacy and gender

O'Donovan and Kirk (2008) suggest that women and girls tend to position themselves around the available discourses in a wide physical and popular culture. Teenage girls, for example, drop out of physical activity at a greater rate than boys, which is an issue that has been evident over the past 50 years without any real change. Reasons girls and teenagers give for dropping out include lack of female role models, greater recognition of boys in sport, and social pressures that sport does not fit with expected images of girls. In general, girls report greater 'body' image dissatisfaction than males, with the result that the more self-conscious girls feel about their 'bodies' the less likely they are to take part in physical activity or sport. As such all those involved in supporting young girls' access to physical activity should be aware of a range of issues concerned with encouraging girls to take part in physical activity. They should promote participation in physical activity as acceptable for girls and challenge gender stereotypes that suggest it is unfeminine to be physically active. They should be aware of girls' self-consciousness about exposing their 'bodies' in a relatively public setting, and ensure that they feel comfortable in their kit. In addition, there is value in ensuring that the range of activities offered is in line with girls' interests.

Case study 12.1 shows clearly that girls in one school were experiencing barriers to taking part in physical activity. Teachers were seen to be unsympathetic, pupils felt uncomfortable both about being seen by others when they were active and because of having to wear unbecoming kit. In addition, the activities they were expected to take part in were not those they would have chosen. Overall there was resistance to physical activity. Girls were losing motivation, their self-esteem and self-confidence were deteriorating and there was no positive development in their physical competence. In short, the girls were making no progress in respect of physical literacy.

Case study 12.1 Girls' attitudes towards school sport

This sports college is a fairly typical mixed, inner-city, 11 to 16 school with relatively challenging socio-economic circumstances. Before this study began, girls were 'very negative' towards physical education (PE) and school sport (PESS), they did not enjoy it, had 'poor relationships' with the staff and physical literacy was generally poor. Girls reported that staff were unhelpful, made no effort to understand their point of view and were generally unsympathetic. A new Head of Girls physical education arrived and decided to work with an inclusion consultant to try to break down some of the barriers preventing girls from taking part in, enjoying and achieving in PESS.

On the back of the results from a forum held with Year 8 and 9 girls several actions were taken including the following:

- A Girls' Sports Council was established where students from Years 7 to 10 communicate ideas for change from across their year groups. Members of staff show their commitment to change by promising to action at least one agreed change by the time of the next meeting.
- A new kit was designed including a choice in style of tracksuit bottoms and the old PE jumper was replaced by a very popular new fleecy hooded top with the school name across the back.
- 'PE pathways' were introduced to Key Stage 4 options, meaning that students now choose a certain route at the beginning of the year according to their own preferences (e.g. fitness, games, dance), but staff can still ensure a balanced programme over the year. Year 9s can now choose from a games and an athletic pathway.

- The old-style gymnasium was converted into a dance/fitness studio with fitness equipment, mirrors, a sound system and no windows (to ensure privacy for the girls).
- Alongside this work there has been a concerted effort among the female PE staff to improve student–staff relations and certain principles run through the success of the concrete actions above. They include better communication, increased respect, higher expectations and a greater commitment to action/change.

The results that these more subtle changes have brought, alongside the concrete changes listed above, are considerable. The girls *themselves* are showing better communication, increased respect, higher expectations and a greater commitment to action/change. The changing room is now a more relaxed place to be, there are fewer excuse notes and girls are getting changed quicker. Lessons are more active, more productive and of a higher standard. After-school clubs have expanded and total numbers taking part exceed those of the boys!

Thus, as a result of listening to their issues and fulfilling promises, teachers have helped to raise these girls' levels of physically literacy by ensuring that they become 'much happier and more confident in the PE department'.[1]

Becoming physically literate can also be difficult for boys (Light 2008) who, for whatever reason, do not match up to the extrovert mesomorph male stereotype. Thus, boys who do not follow traditional physical activity roles and/or take up activities such as dance may find themselves isolated or subject to prejudice. In this regard some schools have established All Boys Dance Clubs to address this problem and minimise feelings of isolation and difference. Furthermore, a wider range of activity opportunities in and out of school could go a long way towards challenging existing patterns of delivery for boys and girls.

Whitehead (2007b, 2007c) also argues that such is the influence of Western patriarchal culture the development of physical literacy by girls and young women has become problematic. Whitehead continues by suggesting that this is due to the way in which male hegemony operates to emphasise the lesser capacity of the embodied dimension of women, alongside attempts to devalue the development of physical competence as unfeminine. It is not surprising that girls and women feel disenfranchised in the current world of sport and physical activity. Internationally, women are under-represented in decision-making positions in physical activity organisations and, according to the Women's Physical Activity and Fitness Foundation (2008), media coverage of physical activity focuses almost entirely on the activities of men. In fact, only around 5 per cent of physical activity coverage in national and local print media within the United Kingdom is dedicated to women's physical activity. As a consequence of this under-representation, physically active women suffer from reduced media coverage and marginalised profiles. Furthermore, what is covered in the media is focused more often on sportswomen's personal lives and/or of these women as objects of desire rather than serious reporting of their physical activity performances and achievements (King 2007). There is an urgent need for the media and physical activity organisations to take proactive steps to develop and support a range of positive female role models as well as seek strategies to raise the 'voice' of women in physical activity, in positions of influence in organisations.

The marginalisation of girls and women in all aspects of physical activity is an issue that has been identified by the Women's Sport and Fitness Foundation (2008). Indeed, the Foundation has noted that only four of the 35 British National governing Bodies of Sport are specifically for women; while only one in four elite coaches are women. The Foundation makes it clear that equality in respect of participation in physical activity and opportunities to become physically literate is not just an issue for young girls; it is a problem that has an ongoing impact throughout life and into adulthood.

In this context the Women's Sport and Fitness Foundation (2008) has identified three core issues that need to be addressed if current inequalities in physical activity are to be addressed. These are seen as vital starting points in measures to rebalance existing gender divides. These are to address:

- the lack of female leaders at the top level of sport
- the inequality of investment both from private and public funds
- the poor promotion of women's sport – both by the media and itself.

Gibbons and Humbert (2008) support such a move in the drive for what they describe as 'an emerging sense of gender equity'. They suggest that, following discussion with women and girls regarding their experiences of physical activity, the key themes to address are those of personal competence, recognition that a moving 'body' is a healthy 'body' and availability of choice and variety of physical activity throughout the lifecourse (Weiss 1999; Kasser and Lytle 2005).

Physical literacy and sexual orientation

Discrimination and/or harassment on the grounds of sexual orientation may not be an immediate consideration for those responsible for physical activity (Connell 2008) but there are occasions in which these attitudes can lessen opportunities for individuals to take part in physical activity and, as a consequence, their ability to realise physical literacy is limited. Homophobia is not acceptable within the modern world and those involved in physical activity have a responsibility to respect this. The types of incidents that may be observed include 'friendly banter', joking and/or verbal/physical violence. Moreover, in the modern world people should not feel that they have to hide their sexual orientation. It is a sad fact that not many physically active men and women in the public arena are open about their sexuality. This limits the opportunity to promote positive role models of gay, lesbian and bisexual individuals (Weeks *et al.* 2003), as often they are concerned that in openly declaring their sexuality they may be subject to prejudice and isolation. Le Blanc and Jackson (2007) note that to date only three gay male athletes have ever come out publicly during their professional physical activity career in team physical activity. This reflects the pervasiveness of homophobia in physical activity and its power to silence and render invisible gay athletes.

Homophobia incorporates irrational fears and intolerance of homosexuality, gay men or lesbians, as well as behaviour that is perceived to be outside the boundaries of traditional gender role expectations. In today's modern world, lesbian, bisexual and gay athletes and coaches should be able to identify themselves if they so choose, without fear of negative consequences. However, the Council of Europe (2003) suggests that physical activity is still considered a masculine domain in Western Europe. Therefore, girls and women who do extremely well in physical activity are seen as threats to existing gender systems which insist on an unequal social construction of womanhood and manhood. Thus, when women enter a 'male' playing field and the female athlete's appearance differs from the feminine stereotype, there is a real chance that she is labelled 'lesbian'. This whole situation leads to a number of important sociological, political, moral and philosophical questions which concern enabling all to have full access to physical activity opportunities. Thus, in relation to homophobia physical activity organisations need to address the need for diversity training with physical activity practitioners and with participants in order to establish progressive and supporting opportunities for all individuals, regardless of their sexual orientation. All individuals should have equal access to participation in physical activity and thus be in a position to develop and maintain physical literacy. Wellard (2009) has written widely on the topic of sport and masculinity, and his insights are valuable.[2]

Physical literacy, religion, faith, race and culture

Family and cultural expectations among certain groups and communities can also have a detrimental impact on individuals' opportunities to develop physical literacy. For example, some cultural practices prohibit exposure of the female 'body' while others consider boys and girls taking up careers or competition in physical activity as a 'waste of time'. Thus, for young people, family and cultural pressures can be very restricting on their attempts to become physically active and thus physically literate. Furthermore, once into adulthood, these young people may reinforce cultural stereotypes with their children unless they are supported and encouraged to challenge existing barriers and restrictions to physical activity.

An individual's cultural practices can be a limiting factor in accessing physical activities of their choice. This may occur as a result of attitudes endemic to particular traditional norms in a country or as the outcome of insensitivity on the part of those organising physical activity in a multicultural setting. Wherever possible, physical activity organisations in these settings and those in positions of authority should take steps to identify any possible instances of indirect discrimination on the grounds of cultural practices that may prevent people from taking part in physical activity. For example, holding all activity sessions or competitions on a Sunday would indirectly discriminate against people from the Christian faith who would wish to attend church. It would be good practice therefore to explore whether some activity sessions or competitions could possibly be held on alternative days.

It is also important for physical activity organisations to understand that an individual should not have to choose between cultural practices and taking part in physical activity. In many religions, a person's faith or belief and thus belonging to a specific community is as much a part of the individual's identity as is his or her gender, ethnic origin or sexual orientation. Indeed, some activities may indirectly minimise opportunities for individuals to access them due to a lack of appreciation of individuals' religious and/or faith needs. For example, Muslim women who wish to take part in swimming activities may need separate sessions with only female coaches and life guards in order to respect their particular need. Failure by organisations to adopt such strategies will, according to Khanifar *et al.* (2008), naturally limit opportunities for participation and engagement with particular activities and in doing so limit opportunities for individuals to develop physical competence and thus physical literacy.

On occasions, assumptions may be made about black and minority ethnic individuals in relation to activities they wish to access. For example, a belief that Asian people do not play football, or that Afro-Caribbean people are good at athletics and basketball, can limit their opportunities to take up a particular physical activity or to participate in a wide range of physical activities. Furthermore, attitudes to women's and girls' embodiment differ in different cultures and religions. The religious and cultural requirements of some Muslim girls and women concerning 'body' modesty may prevent them from appearing in front of men, dressed in inappropriate attire. This is just one of the factors which results in lower than average participation rates in certain activities. Thus, if organisations show respect for racial and cultural diversity and take positive steps to consult and negotiate with individuals, positive strides forward can be made to increase opportunities for everyone to engage in physical activity.

Case study 12.2 outlines a piece of research carried put in Birmingham (Benn *et al.* 2009; Dagkas *et al.* 2009). It shows how, with thought, consultation and flexibility, opportunities for physical activity can be enhanced.

Case study 12.2 A solution to intercultural tensions

An example of partnership in seeking a solution to intercultural tensions may be seen from a recent project carried out in England, in a large multiethnic city with many different religions, the largest minority group being Pakistani and Muslim. The problem arose when Muslim parents started withdrawing their daughters from physical education lessons on religious grounds.

In relation to physical education, the religiosity of some Muslim families led to preferences to 'embody faith' in ways that were denied in the traditional systems and structures of physical education and sports participation in England. Preferences related to body modesty, covering arms, legs and head, and gender segregation which were considered essential for some, not least to identify Muslim women. Traditional cultural expectations in England in physical education and school sport such as mixed-sex lessons and shorts and T-shirts were barriers to participation by these families, hence the withdrawal. The problem was not with participating in physical activity but with the systems and structures that denied preferences to embody faith.

Headteachers were sometimes unable to meet requests to change policy and practice, often for pragmatic reasons such as same-sex staffing if groups were split or pool environments were being managed by local leisure services and therefore beyond their control. As a result of a research project, in which there was wide consultation with schools and families, good practice features were identified from some schools, documented and then shared as guidance. Common to these were principles of flexibility, respect for personal choice and accommodation of difference. The emphasis was on making changes to be more inclusive. The most important point was giving students access to participation in physical activity. In schools, least difficulty arose where parents were fully informed of expectations and strong links had been developed between the school and the families.

Young people whose schools and families had been involved in the consultations and debates report enthusiastically on the effect this has had on their opportunities to take part in a range of physical activities within and beyond the curriculum. These young people appreciated the way they had been involved in the discussions and the respect that had been shown to the traditions within their various cultures.[3]

Strategies to support diversity in physical literacy

Vickerman (2007) suggests that in order to offer equality of opportunity in physical activity and consequently furtherance of physical literacy, a range of strategies need to be adopted. All those responsible for mounting and leading physical activity need to be challenged to think flexibly and openly about the diversity of methods they must adopt to minimise barriers to physical activity. In doing so an 'Eight P' Inclusive Framework (Vickerman 2007) is proposed to encourage all those involved in facilitating inclusive physical activity to undertake a full and detailed review of what needs to be considered to meet the full diversity of individuals' needs.

In considering this framework the first feature is a need to appreciate the *philosophy* of inclusive physical activity and its relationships to basic and fundamental human rights. This requires consideration of how human rights are supported as a society through statutory and non-statutory guidance and principles of the International Salamanca Statement (UNESCO 1994) and UN and EU declarations noted earlier within this chapter. It therefore requires those involved in facilitating physical activity to understand the philosophical basis and principles of inclusion as well as buying into the notion that all individuals, regardless of their gender, sexual orientation, race, culture or faith, have a fundamental entitlement to realise their potential with respect to physical literacy.

In order to acknowledge the philosophical complexities of inclusion, a *purposeful* approach (Fredrickson and Cline 2002) to fulfilling the requirements of inclusive physical activity should be considered. By examining various philosophical standpoints a clear appreciation of the rationale and arguments behind the inclusive strategies may be understood and the way forward to provide positive movement experiences for all identified.

In order to achieve this, all stakeholders must be *proactive* in the development, implementation and review of inclusive activity (Centre for Studies in Inclusive Education 2008). They should be prepared to work in *partnership* and consult actively with groups and individuals from diverse backgrounds in order to maximise an appreciation of how to minimise barriers to physical activity. In addition, inclusive activity necessitates a commitment to modify, adapt and change existing strategies, policies and practices in order to facilitate full access and entitlement. This must be recognised as part of a *process* model that evolves, emerges and changes over time, and as such needs regular review and reflection.

Inclusive physical activity is also now reflected internationally within *policy* and legislative documentation. This sets out to state publicly how agencies are going to respond to inclusive practice, while also being used as a means of holding people to account (UN 2008). Those managing physical activity, however, must recognise the need to move policies through into their *pedagogical* practices in order to ensure that practitioners have the necessary skills (Rink and Hall 2008) to deliver inclusive physical activity. Consequently, while philosophies and processes are vital, they must in due course be measured in terms of effective and successful inclusive *practice* that values person-centred approaches to the learning and development of everyone.

Conclusion: the universality of physical literacy

This chapter has set out to assert that physical literacy is a universal concept which can be attained by every human being where the right opportunities are provided. Whitehead (2007d) suggests that as human beings we all experience the world from an embodied (Gibbs 2006) perspective, bringing our unique nature to this interaction. Difference and diversity enrich all our lives and influence attitudes to, and experiences of, physical activity. However, differences must be accommodated fully and flexibly if opportunities are to be offered to everyone to engage in physical activity and to grow in physical competence (Cole 2008).

All stakeholders need to show genuine empathy to the full range of diversity of individuals within society. Those who have characteristics that single them out as different with respect to, for example, gender, sexual orientation, race, culture and religion must have the same opportunities to be involved in physical activity and thus to realise and maintain physical literacy. All individuals should be accommodated, limitations minimised and barriers surmounted This will only be achieved by practitioners, both in positions of power and involved in delivery, adopting proactive strategies and having open minds to think flexibly about how diversity can be celebrated, rather than seen as a restriction on access to gaining positive physical activity experiences.

Recommended reading

Norwich, B. (2002) Education, inclusion and individual differences: recognising and resolving dilemmas. *British Journal of Education Studies*, 50, 4, pp. 482–502.
    This research paper provides a useful insight into strategies to identify and resolve differences among individuals and groups. The paper identifies how inclusion policy and practice has developed within the United Kingdom and the issues this brings in meeting individual needs.

Whitehead, M.E. (2007a) Physical Literacy and its importance to every individual. National Association for Disability, Dublin, Ireland, January. Available on the website www.physical-literacy.org.uk.
    This paper provides a comprehensive overview of the needs of a range of individuals and the potential to limit and/or address their access to physical literacy. The paper will be useful for anyone supporting diverse groups and individuals in reflecting upon strategies for minimising barriers to access and participation in physical activity.

Part III
Practical implications

13 Promoting physical literacy within and beyond the school curriculum

Margaret Whitehead

Introduction

This chapter will briefly review Part I and Part II and will then consider some aspects of the promotion of physical literacy within and beyond the school setting. Issues covered will include the role of significant others in fostering and maintaining physical literacy, including physical education teachers. The relationship between physical literacy, physical activity and physical education will then be explained. The chapter will lay the ground for Chapter 14 which looks at learning and teaching approaches in the context of nurturing physical literacy, and Chapter 15 which is concerned to present a case for involving individuals in a wide range of physical activities.

Areas discussed in Part I and Part II

Part I set out the concept of physical literacy and outlined the rationale behind the different elements of the concept, with reference to the philosophical underpinning, as appropriate. Part II considered ways in which physical literacy connects with issues in a range of specific contexts such as the physical self and the rise in levels of obesity. The importance of physical literacy to the young child and the older adult population was discussed, as were the benefits of, and barriers to, physical literacy for particular populations. Before considering some of the practical implications of the concept of physical literacy with reference to the range of practices and personnel involved, it will be helpful to draw together, briefly, the key points that have been debated in the foregoing text.

Physical literacy is founded on monist principles that see the individual human being as one indivisible whole. As human beings, individuals have a range of different constituent dimensions each of which generates a human capability. These capabilities, while they can be discussed separately, are never experienced discretely by the individual. The capabilities are intricately interrelated and interdependent, which means that employment or development of any of these has an effect on the totality of the person. In line with this view, as has been outlined, are the ways in which development of our embodied capability can contribute to linguistic, cognitive, rational and emotional development. An individual's sense of self is built up through experience of drawing on these irrevocably interconnected capabilities. There is no doubt that effective deployment of our embodied capability can make a positive contribution to self-perception and self-esteem, as well as to confidence in self-presentation and effective relationships with others.

Physical literacy is also founded on the view that individuals are essentially beings-in-the-world who create themselves through interaction with their environment. In this context those aspects of our human condition through which we can make contact with the world have particular significance. Our embodied dimension is one such aspect and is therefore a key aspect of our personhood.

The study of existentialism and phenomenology revealed a significant role for our embodied dimension and the capability this generates. The nature of this capability was seen to go beyond commonly used descriptions of embodied ability such as being able to move skilfully and being physically educated. In order to highlight the perceptions of these schools of philosophy a term that referred specifically to our embodied capability was needed. The term identified was physical literacy. This term goes beyond the use of our embodied dimension as a tool or mechanism and incorporates the involvement of this dimension as lived. The notion of the 'body', which, in the English language, is only associated with this human dimension as an object, is not felt to be helpful, and thus the dimension is referred to as the embodied dimension rather than the 'body'. The embodied dimension encompasses both the embodiment-as-lived and the embodiment-as-instrument.

Physical literacy as a human capability is pertinent to all individuals whenever and wherever they live and whatever age they are. The capability, though relevant to all individuals, is also specific to each individual, reflecting both their unique endowment and the cultural context within which they live. While a broad progressive outline of achieving the attributes of physical literacy, including embodied competences, can be described, the normative grading of individuals and thus comparison with 'expectations' and with others is inappropriate. Individuals' development and their step-by-step mastery is where the focus should lie. The charting of individual progress, recording and rewarding mastery, however small, is the most appropriate approach to any form of assessment. Individuals will have their own personal potential and must be respected as unique. Any assessment must, therefore, be in the form of charting the progress each is making on their personal and unique journey to becoming physically literate.

Physical literacy and significant others

As discussed by Whitehead with Murdoch (2006), the development and maintenance of physical literacy throughout life will be influenced by numerous significant others. These people will be in a position to provide opportunities for physical activity both in the home and beyond. Through their attitudes and reactions to the efforts of participants, they will also play a significant role in affecting how readily those with whom they come into contact become physically literate. While opportunities for activity are critical, a supportive and encouraging attitude towards participants is even more important. Opportunities may change as individuals move from childhood, through adulthood to old age; however, the need for sympathetic encouragement is critical at all ages. The embodied dimension and embodied capability are significant aspects of personhood, self-respect and self-confidence. Insensitive negative comments can easily be taken very personally, with the result that motivation may decrease and participation may cease to be a positive experience. This unfortunate situation can occur at any time from childhood, through adulthood into old age. The result of such negative experiences may well be that involvement in physical activity is not maintained and physical literacy is not attained or developed.

In this context is it valuable to look briefly at each stage in life and identify the role that significant others can play in the development and nurturing of physical literacy.

In the early years until the start of compulsory schooling, the most significant players in the development of physical literacy will be parents or principal carers. As was outlined in Chapter 9, this is a critical stage in establishing the foundations of physical literacy. Parents or carers should be encouraged to give these young children plenty of opportunities to move about and exercise in the home and outdoors. Large movements involving the whole embodied dimension such as running, jumping and climbing should be encouraged as well as challenges demanding dexterity such as turning the pages of a book, managing a knife, fork and spoon, and throwing and catching a ball. There should be ample opportunities for free play, guided play and structured play. At all times the parent or carer should be enthusiastic and supportive. Other significant players at this stage may include nursery nurses, day care personnel and teachers and coaches running activity sessions for young children. It is important that all these practitioners offer opportunities in a wide range of activities, show excitement in response to progress and effort, and give positive feedback. All significant individuals in contact with young children need to provide environments that offer openings for exploration but are at the same time safe. As young children experiment in the movement context, carers and practitioners should guard against being too cautious or in any way indicating that the activity is risky and may cause harm. In the early years children are very aware of the attitudes of adults, and if they sense nervousness they are likely to be apprehensive, lose confidence and be far less inquisitive and adventurous. The establishment of enjoyment in the movement context is critical for the development of physical literacy.

When the child moves into compulsory schooling a new group of significant others are brought into play. These are teachers. The key role that these significant others play in the development and fostering of physical literacy cannot be stressed too strongly. These teachers play a very important part for at least four reasons. First, they provide the only guaranteed opportunity for all children to develop their embodied competence; second, these teachers will have expertise in working with children and young adults and, particularly in respect of teachers of the older age groups, will have good knowledge and understanding of movement. In addition, teachers will have access to a wide range of activity settings and be able to provide a rich variety of experiences for young people. Finally, teachers are often held in some esteem by their students, and their views can be very influential in the development of attitudes that these young people acquire.

With reference to the younger age groups it is critical that teachers maintain the natural exuberance that most children exhibit in respect of physical activity. This is challenging, as in many cases the teacher will be responsible for all areas of learning, will not be a physical education specialist and may not have had the opportunity to acquire a great deal of knowledge and understanding of children's movement. At the very least these teachers should provide experience of a range of physical activities, promote all-round movement competence and ensure that every child is working at an appropriate level, achieving success which is recognised and applauded. There should be no sense of failure and minimal comparison with the work of other pupils. These young people should be accepted as individuals, each with their strengths and each able to move forward in their development of physical literacy. Confidence and motivation must be sustained.

Those teachers working with older age groups, very often physical education specialists, have the same responsibilities but their task is much more challenging. While young children have a natural love for movement activity, as they mature through to adolescence not only do they have to manage their growing and changing physical selves, they are very much influenced by cultural expectations. As was seen in Chapter 12, this can be a particular problem for girls and some young people from particular ethnic backgrounds. Teachers need to be sensitive to cultural pressures, whether from peers or family. Nevertheless, it is incumbent on the teachers to enable all pupils to achieve and further their physical literacy. Not only should a wide variety of activities be offered but the teaching must be planned and presented so that every young person is successful and receives praise and recognition for their progress.

All teachers, both generalist in earlier education and specialist in later education, should understand the importance and value of physical literacy and realise that their work in the school curriculum is critical, being the most focused and highly developed context in which this capability can be established, fostered and celebrated.

Alongside teachers there are a wide range of other significant individuals who can play a part in promoting a positive attitude to physical activity and thus to fostering physical literacy during the years of schooling. The opportunities that parents and carers provide continue to be significant, as are their attitudes towards physical activity. Other family members and peers play a part in developing activity patterns and shaping views as to the value of physical activity. In addition, practitioners working in extra-curricular contexts at school or beyond have a key role to play, as do paramedical personnel in contact with pupils with disabilities. It is essential that all these practitioners interact with participants as individuals and have these young people at the forefront of planning and guidance. The underlying approach to the work must be teaching the young people rather than teaching the activity. All those involved in working with children and young people must do all they can to promote a positive attitude towards physical activity and to guard against any feelings of failure on the part of the participant. While reference to sports stars and other high-level performers can be inspirational for some, this can also result in those who do not have exceptional potential perceiving that physical activity is not for them. These pupils, in realising that they can never reach such amazing levels of skill, may well lose motivation and withdraw from participation in physical activity as soon as they can. That young people leave compulsory schooling physically literate is critical. Importantly, all significant others at this stage of life should share the same goal of developing physical literacy. This will be evidenced in the attitudes these practitioners show and the manner in which they interact with young people. Young people's perception of physical activity and their attitude to participation tend to be established in these formative years and, as was discussed in Chapter 7, can be very hard to change. Where motivation, confidence and physical competence is well established there is a strong possibility that physical literacy will be maintained throughout the lifecourse, with the potential of significant life-enriching experiences.

While it is hoped that, on leaving school, individuals will be physically literate and thus have a robust and positive attitude to physical activity and be self motivated to continue participation, a new set of circumstances and significant others come into play. Involvement in physical activity will now have to be woven into patterns of work and family responsibilities. There may also be issues of cost. In addition, the attitudes of family, friends and colleagues may influence participation. It is important that all of these influential individuals appreciate the importance and value of maintaining physical literacy and are supportive of continued participation. Where negative views are repeatedly and forcefully expressed either about the value of physical activity or the embodied competences with which a person is endowed it may be difficult or impossible for participation to continue. Where participation is maintained it will be important for those managing the activity to be welcoming and supportive to all. Those in positions of responsibility in clubs, classes and leisure centres will be particularly influential and their acceptance of the efforts of every individual will be crucial if younger and older adults are to persevere with current activities, reassess their abilities, try new activities as appropriate, and learn new skills that are in tune with their competence as they grow older.

As the adult reaches old age the importance of physical literacy is likely to increase rather than decrease and the benefits can be significant, as has been outlined in Chapter 10. However, this group of the population may be very hard to motivate to become involved in physical activity. Some of these individuals may have been active but have ceased to take much exercise in later life, others may never have been regularly involved in physical activity and yet others may have entrenched negative feelings towards activity that have developed at some time in the past. A consistent and positive attitude towards participation needs to be evident among all significant others including family, friends, carers, medical and paramedical personnel and staff in leisure centres. Opportunities for physical activity need to be available and steps taken to enable all older people to take part. As before, all those managing and supporting these activities need to be encouraging and enthusiastic. There is little doubt that older people who are physically literate live a fuller, healthier and often longer life.

The expectations identified above with respect to the role that significant others can play in promoting physical activity depend to a great extent on the opportunities and facilities that are available in the local area. In this respect a great deal of responsibility for fostering physical literacy throughout the lifecourse rests with policy-makers in central and local government, those in executive positions in governing bodies of sport and other forms of physical activity, and those managing health centres, leisure centres and clubs. Without the appropriate investment and strategic management of resources, little progress will be made in respect of the goal to enable all to achieve and maintain physical literacy.

The contribution of significant others, particularly teachers and other adults such as coaches and sports club and leisure centre personnel, is critical in developing physical literacy, and thus Chapters 14 and 15 are devoted to examining aspects of their contribution in detail. However, prior to these discussions it will be valuable to clarify the relationship between physical literacy, physical activity and physical education.

Fostering and maintaining physical literacy as the goal of physical activity and physical education

There would seem a strong case to argue that for all those in positions to encourage, organise or lead physical activity, the development and fostering of physical literacy is the underlying goal of the enterprise. There is a close relationship between physical activity and physical education and the concept of physical literacy. However, they are of a different order. Physical activity and physical education are situations in which participants are active. Physical literacy is a goal or aspiration in respect of the outcome of these situations. Physical activity and physical education are 'events', while physical literacy is characterised by the development of a disposition in participants. Indeed, the promotion and development of physical literacy can be seen as describing the value of physical activity: a value that can be supported and justified philosophically and scientifically, as detailed in Part I.

Far from calling into question or contesting current aspirations in relation to physical activity and physical education, and far from being in competition with many of the often cited values for this work, physical literacy sets out a clear direction for practitioners leading physical activity. The concept of physical literacy draws together and brings coherence to the wide range of views in respect of the value of participation in physical activity. For example, the aims concerning experiencing enjoyment, developing independence, mastering physical skills, learning to work with others and appreciating the concept of health-related fitness are all integral to the concept.

A very significant aspect of physical literacy is the identification of the intrinsic and unique value of this capability, arising as it does from our embodied dimension. Physical literacy is a fundamental human capability, indispensable to the way in which human beings create themselves and conduct their lives. It is in the interests of each individual to develop this capability – indeed it is the responsibility of each culture to ensure that physical literacy is nurtured in all members of society. Establishment of this capability creates a sound platform for lifelong participation in physical activity and provides an ideal springboard for those who have exceptional potential with respect to this capability.

In identifying the goal of physical activity and physical education as developing physical literacy, the credentials of which may be clearly articulated, the professionals involved in this field will no longer need to argue for the place of this work as a means to other ends. Work that focuses on the embodied dimension is of value in its own right. In addition, these practitioners can rebuff criticisms that label physical activity as purely recreational, and thus trivial and peripheral to 'serious' education in the broadest sense. Furthermore, the concept, as it applies throughout life, establishes a scenario in which there are many players involved in promoting physical literacy. While teachers play the key role they must be supported by numerous others from, for example, the family, the medical profession and the government.

Physical literacy in no way undermines physical education or coaching. The concept is not in competition with physical education; rather, it is enormously supportive of this area of work. Physical literacy offers the opportunity for all involved in promoting physical activity to speak with one voice, to articulate a clear goal, and furthermore to make a strong case for every pupil to have the opportunity to develop this capability. Every individual should have the opportunity to express and develop their physical literacy, not only to realise their human potential but also to enhance their quality of life.

Chapter 14 discusses how support and teaching might be conducted to promote the development and maintenance of physical literacy, and Chapter 15 considers how a breadth of experience in different activity settings is essential to participants achieving all the attributes of physical literacy.

Recommended reading

Whitehead, M.E. with Murdoch, E. (2006) Physical literacy and physical education: conceptual mapping. *Physical Education Matters*, Summer.

14 Physical literacy and learning and teaching approaches

Dominic Haydn-Davies

Introduction

This chapter outlines how learning can be structured to develop physical literacy. It aims to relate the philosophical and theoretical aspects of earlier chapters to practice. The discussion focuses on learning and teaching approaches to promote physical literacy. The chapter aims to demonstrate how a range of aspects of teaching can be used effectively to develop physical literacy and to suggest that *how* teaching is conducted is as important, or possibly more important, than *what* is taught.

When aiming to develop physical literacy in participants it is vital that these individuals are the central focus of any teaching approach. As a practitioner, the decision to employ a particular teaching approach should spring from the needs of the participants: learner first, learning next, with the activity being the context for that learning. It is this decision that is of fundamental importance to any teaching that aims to develop physical literacy.

The practitioner is understood to refer to any individual who is organising, managing and overseeing physical activity. This individual could be, for example, a teacher, coach, sports development officer, parent or paramedic.

Any learning/teaching interaction needs to have motivation at its core. For participants to develop physical literacy they need to feel confident about their potential for progress and success. Every interaction should strive to maintain or increase motivation wherever possible. Even when temporary loss of motivation is apparent, all aspects of teaching must remain positive, being responsive and proactive, highlighting where next steps to learning can be achieved. Motivation is the key to physical literacy and therefore needs to be the central driver when choices are made about teaching. In addition, all approaches need to build towards developing self-confidence, self-esteem and self-respect. Where any of these are threatened, motivation is likely to decrease, commitment to participate may deteriorate, and as a result physical literacy will not be established or enhanced.

Interaction between practitioner and participant

The key focus of the interaction – be it teacher–child; coach–athlete; carer–adult; parent–child – must be to answer the question: How do I motivate and enable individuals to capitalise on and build from what they can do? Answers will need to take into consideration factors relating to the extent and breadth of experience of the participants and the nature of the environment, including other people in the activity setting. As a practitioner aiming to foster positive development of an individual's physical literacy there is a variety of other factors that need to be considered explicitly. The biggest challenge, for most, arises from the embodied nature of each individual. Individuals need to be seen as more than just 'bodies' to be 'trained'; they are complex, embodied human beings. Their development and progress will not be linear or always continuous. The skilled and sensitive practitioner should expect, accept and respect differences. As far as possible, differences should be seen as expressions of individual characteristics and abilities rather than in a hierarchical context in comparison with those of others. It is clear that to develop physical literacy in an individual, the practitioner needs at all times to be aspiring to and anticipating progress and success on the part of each learner. There is no one-size-fits-all approach. It is important that it is acknowledged that 'every individual is different, will confront a given task in their own unique way and will adapt to the environment they are working in differently to others' (Pickup and Price 2007: 29).

To develop physical literacy an individual would need to experience a range of activities, challenges and opportunities as detailed in Chapter 15. These form the 'what' for the practitioner. The focus of this chapter is on something possibly more important – 'how' participation in these activities is managed to ensure that physical literacy remains at the heart of the enterprise. Three key factors are profiled in more detail: the climate of the interaction, the qualities of the practitioner and the teaching skills employed.

Climate of the interaction

The climate of a session refers to the ambience or 'feeling' of the overall interaction. This is created by a combination of management, monitoring and maintenance. The climate looks beyond the physical environment to the perceptions and responses of individuals and groups in the context of the range of interactions and features that are part of the experience. Importantly, any session should evolve so that all participants feel they are valued, experience progress and thus retain and/or establish motivation whatever the setting.

All participants will have different reasons and motivations for taking part in the activity and some of these may seem less than helpful in promoting physical literacy. For example, anxiety or fear are common feelings when starting a new activity. These feelings may appear problematic as elements of individuals' motivation; however, if participants can use this apprehension to spur them on to engage in the new activity and overcome challenges, then there is no reason why individuals cannot progress and maintain motivation. However, while in some circumstances it may be possible to capitalise on and channel anxiety, fear of punishment or exclusion must not be used as planned motivational devices in working to develop physical literacy. Similarly, both pressure to participate in the context of an undue risk of injury and pressure to conform to social stereotypes, without regard for the individual's own identity, should be avoided. Such pressures are highly likely to be counter-productive in working to promote motivation and confidence and thus physical literacy.

Climate maintenance is an ongoing process of negotiation and adaptability. The climate needs to promote, not hinder progress. To establish and maintain a positive, supporting ambience the practitioner will clearly need certain personal qualities and be able to use a variety of appropriate skills and teaching strategies.

Qualities and teaching skills of the practitioner

The practitioner who aims to develop physical literacy in every member of a group has a challenging task. It is not necessarily as simple as having good knowledge of particular activities, or being a good organiser, or even being able to relate to individuals. A practitioner may have a particular 'strength' in one or more of these categories, but must be willing and able to adapt and apply these attributes in the interests of the participants. So while practitioners will need sound practical knowledge and group management skills it is perhaps the qualities they display that will be most important. Significant among these qualities will be sensitivity, empathy, patience, appreciation of effort and an encouraging and enthusiastic approach to the work. Practitioners need to have well-developed non-verbal communication skills such as self-presentation, posture, gesture and facial expressions. They should communicate effectively with individuals, using the most appropriate and clear form of communication available. They should recognise and applaud effort, application, progress and achievement in equal measure. They should aim to give regular and focused praise, encouragement and informative feedback. As with any relationship, they should respect the participants and what each brings to the interaction. Using participants' names is not only a sign of this respect but also a confirmation that the practitioner knows each participant as an individual. At all times practitioners should demonstrate a positive attitude towards participants and a sincere interest in the interaction. In addition, interactions between practitioner and participant need to be understood in terms of an ongoing relationship with all the ethical and moral responsibilities this may bring.

As mentioned earlier, there are numerous aspects or skills of teaching that can be used by practitioners to help individuals progress towards their potential in respect of developing physical literacy. What is important is that these aspects or 'tools' are chosen carefully and used in a skilful and appropriate way.

To promote physical literacy, decisions have to be taken in planning and delivering a session in respect of a number of dimensions of the teaching, as set out below. It will be valuable to consider the answers to the following questions. The answer to each question will signpost the need to use certain teaching skills. These skills will cover planning, delivery and evaluation in the context of learning and teaching.

Content selected/planning

- Has the session been planned with the *participant(s)* at the heart of the experience?
- Will the *content* meet the expectations of the participants?
- Are the *tasks* selected appropriate to the participants' abilities and motivation?
- Will there be regular *chances to achieve* and succeed?

Organisation

- Does the *structure* of the session meet the physical, social and emotional needs of the participant(s)?
- Are *timings* planned to suit the participants or have they been imposed from external factors?
- Are there a variety of *resources*, including media, available to support and challenge participants?[1]
- Have the *expectations of behaviour* been agreed?
- Are *rules and routines* negotiated, agreed and well articulated?
- Are organisational *cues* understood?
- Is the *learning environment* safe, stimulating and challenging?

Learning/teaching interaction

- Does the *climate* promote mutual respect between practitioner and participant(s) and between participants?
- Is *feedback* given constructively, frequently and positively?
- Is *assessment for learning* used to promote progress?
- Will the participants understand if they are *improving*?
- Are both *verbal and non-verbal communication* used effectively and regularly?
- Is account taken of *participants' responses* such that tasks are modified appropriately?

- Are *questions* used to support learning and progress?
- Are *participants* encouraged to ask questions?

The answers to these questions challenge the practitioner to call on or develop a variety of teaching skills such as movement observation, time management, phrasing questions in a variety of ways, giving appropriate feedback and effecting sound assessment procedures. Alongside these elements of the interaction the practitioner will need to ensure that the selection of material and resources and the planning of tasks match the needs of the participants.

All these elements of how teaching is carried out are crucial in developing participants' enjoyment, progress and confidence in their involvement in physical activity. The key to practitioners promoting physical literacy is to reflect on interactions that occur in an activity session. A greater awareness of these variables listed above and their impact on participants will enable practitioners to be more reflective, understand the impact different aspects of teaching have on participants and ultimately be more successful in fostering physical literacy. The fundamental concern must always be the participants, their progress and motivation, and the confidence they have in their abilities.

Individual learners

Throughout the book it has been stressed that physical literacy must be seen as a capability the expression of which is unique to the individual. The uniqueness rests on each individual's endowment in respect of all their human dimensions. While physical competence will clearly be important in developing physical literacy, other characteristics such as self-confidence and social skills will also be significant. It is against this background that practitioners need to select the teaching skills or 'tools' they will use. In an ideal situation practitioners can select the 'tools' to match the needs of the individual. Case study 14.1 provides some examples it is valuable to consider. The question is: would the scenarios described provide each participant with opportunities to develop the *'the motivation, confidence, physical competence, knowledge and understanding to maintain physical activity throughout the lifecourse'*?

In considering these scenarios it is useful to identify aspects of the interaction that may inhibit the development of physical literacy. In some cases it may be difficult to decide if the approach will be productive or not. This will be because each participant is unique, with some able to thrive even in less supportive situations and others being very sensitive to comments from, and reactions of, those with whom activity is taking place. Problems will arise where the teaching approach is not well matched to the participant's motivation or ability. The responsibility lies with the practitioners, who should know their participants and plan the interaction in their interests.

Case study 14.1 Scenarios

- Owen, a young child, is taken to his favourite adventure play area and given strict instructions by a new play worker about what he has to do.
- Asa is out playing football with friends in the park. An adult comes and organises them into groups practising skills and passing.
- Maya and her friends are going to their first social dance class. They are told to 'have a go' when they arrive and are not given any instruction.
- Meredith is new to a well-established, high-performing gymnastics group. She is put into a leadership position in her first session.
- Peter goes swimming on his lunch break and has done every week for the past twenty years. Another swimmer keeps challenging him to races and gives feedback on his technique.
- Amelie is starting driving lessons and is told by her instructor to 'see what works for you'.
- Thea and her group of elderly friends meet with an enthusiastic practitioner every week, but he never asks them what they enjoy or what they like.
- Jonty is a high performing athlete. His new coach insists that he goes back to a more traditional type of training. The coach also insists he is called Sir, and never uses his athletes' names – he demands respect.

With respect to each learner, practitioners might consider, for example, the degree of challenge, the nature of the feedback, the social context and the mode of motivation that are likely to be most productive. Above all they must show empathy towards each and every participant. However, as physical literacy is a lifelong disposition there is also the need for participants to begin to take responsibility for their own participation and learning. There is, therefore, another set of possibilities to consider. For example how far are participants ready to:

- select the tasks on which they are to work;
- set the targets towards which they are working;
- evaluate their own performance;
- plan the next step in their learning/activity programme;
- suggest and test their own solutions to problems;
- create tasks rather than follow pre-given instructions.

This list is also important in considering how learning and teaching approaches can support the development of the knowledge and understanding of movement as outlined in the attributes of being physically literate, as discussed in Chapter 6.

Working with groups

The scenarios and lists above provide a real challenge for the practitioner to design and deliver the most effective learning environment for each participant. The situation becomes more difficult when there are groups of participants involved. As this is the most common setting for the nurturing of physical literacy, the challenge of group work needs consideration. The practitioner will need to draw up a session plan that, as far as possible, accommodates the needs of all participants. Just as working with an individual should be specific to that person, so each session plan will be particular to the needs of each group. However, within this overall plan careful thought should be given to, for example:

- how work can be planned so that each participant has real opportunities to experience success;
- in what parts of the session differentiated tasks can be provided;
- in what ways participants can have more or less time to work on a task;
- in what types of social settings can each participant thrive.

Working in groups, while challenging for the practitioner, is very important in developing some of the attributes of physical literacy. It is suggested in Chapter 6 that the physically literate individual has the confidence and abilities to interact effectively with others and can use and read non-verbal messages in this interaction. Group settings within the learning/teaching situation and in activity settings are very valuable in that they give opportunities for working in collaborative and competitive ways, for discussing and sharing issues and for learning to relate sensitively to others.

The session climate, the personal qualities and teaching skills of the practitioner as recommended above apply to all interactions aimed to promote physical literacy. However, the specific nature of the elements of teaching selected will need to be chosen with the particular group in mind. Within this structure practitioners should aspire to cater, as far as possible, for the needs of each individual.

This chapter has focused on generic principles, relevant to the work of all practitioners. However, it is also important to take account of the specific needs of particular populations. This is addressed in some detail in earlier chapters. Chapter 9 looks at work with young children, while Chapter 10 is concerned with promoting physical literacy in the older adult population. Chapters 11 and 12 consider, respectively, those with special needs and issues related to physical literacy and diversity.

Teaching strategies/interaction styles

The notion of teaching strategies or interaction styles will be familiar to most teachers and coaches. However, it will be valuable here to introduce these briefly for the benefit of other practitioners, and to remind those who are aware of these ways of categorising the learning/teaching process how use of different strategies might be valuable in promoting physical literacy. Simply put, a teaching strategy is a cluster of teaching skills that has been selected to achieve a particular outcome, with either an individual learner or a group. A number of writers have suggested different systems of strategies; however, the system devised by Mosston and Ashworth (2002) is particularly useful as it was drawn up with the teaching of physical activity in mind. While the system is not without its critics it provides a useful structure within which to look at broader teaching systems. Mosston and Ashworth's 'spectrum' of styles or strategies is differentiated by the pattern of decision-making within a teaching episode.[2] At one end of their spectrum the practitioner makes nearly all the decisions about what will take place in a session, while at the other end the participant is responsible for all of the decisions. With respect to the knowledge, understanding and mastery achieved in each style, the spectrum is sometimes described as being concerned with replication and reliance on others at one end, and creation and taking responsibility at the other. This development aligns well with the physical literacy journey of each individual, starting with reliance on clear guidance and culminating in taking full responsibility for involvement in physical activity as a lifelong habit/pursuit. Mosston and Ashworth claim that no style is superior to any other but that each is designed to achieve a particular learning outcome. For example, some styles are designed to result in the production of clearly defined movement outcomes while others aspire to support learners to work within their own potential. Some styles work to develop social skills, others to foster the ability to evaluate movement, and others to solve problems and create new movement patterns. The key to selecting an interaction style is to find a match between the style, the group or individual and the intended learning outcomes in question. A particular interaction style does not have to last for the whole of a lesson, nor do all participants in a group have to be working in the same interaction style. Further study of the styles will reveal that each depends on a range of abilities and characteristics of the participants; for example, age, experience, confidence, social skills and independence. It is the case that the use of a range of styles can be very valuable in fostering physical literacy. However, it is also true that an ill-chosen style may hamper progress in one or more of the attributes of physical literacy. The recommendation that practitioners will be more effective if they have mastered a repertoire of teaching strategies or interaction styles is endorsed by Kulinna and Cothran (2003: 579) who assert that a characteristic of an effective practitioner is a 'mastery of multiple teaching styles'. Doherty and Brennan (2008) support this, as would Mosston, who writes (1972: 6): 'the teacher who is familiar with a variety of teaching styles is ready to cope with new conditions and to interact successfully with various forms of student behaviour'.

The notion of being versatile in the teaching situation is also pertinent to the use of teaching skills. The practitioner needs to be able to draw from a wide range of these teaching tools to accommodate, as far as possible, the needs of each group and individual in that group. To suggest that one way of teaching will suit all participants, activities, contexts or participants fails to take into account the complex nature of the embodied human being. The question is not just *which* is best but which is best *when* and for *whom*.

The self-reflective practitioner

While the teaching interaction to promote physical literacy can be set out simply, with its focus on responding to individuals and groups, its demands to be ever encouraging and positive and its reliance on sensitivity and empathy at all times, the mastery of these aspects of teaching is challenging. The development of a repertoire of skills and strategies will take time, as will the ability to select the best way to interact with participants. The ability to be engaged in a continuous process of refining and expanding this repertoire is a key factor when aiming to become a more effective practitioner.

This mastery may be seen as a process, acquired over time, through astute observation, honest self-reflection and constructive self-criticism. The process relies on the practitioner's willingness and ability to reflect, learn, adapt, and remain committed to promoting physical literacy. This development will be enhanced and enriched by engaging in purposeful dialogue with participants and with other practitioners. As work is carried out with individuals and groups the characteristics of these participants will change. It is therefore the case that the practitioner will need to review teaching frequently to cater for these changes.

Conclusion

Physical literacy is pertinent throughout life. In essence it is a disposition, rather than a product or a process. Nevertheless enhancing physical literacy should be the product or outcome of any involvement in physical activity and this ongoing enhancement may be seen as a process. The fostering of this process is in the hands of all those practitioners with whom the individual comes into contact. Working with a range of participants in a variety of contexts and environments will provide invaluable experiences for practitioners, and reflecting on these will enable them to react and adapt to new situations more readily. The reflection should focus on the participants involved and on how effective the learning/teaching approaches have been. This is demanding for the practitioners, as every learner is unique and will need particular tasks and feedback to foster the development of physical literacy.

A practitioner aiming to develop physical literacy will aspire to:

- understand the key principles and philosophies of physical literacy and adopt these as central to their values and beliefs;
- develop participants' motivation, confidence, physical competence, knowledge and understanding to maintain physical activity, as appropriate to their individual endowment, throughout the lifecourse;
- be patient, caring and empathetic as well as challenging and demanding, and set high standards at all times;
- understand the implications of their practice on all the attributes of physical literacy;
- reflect critically and constructively on all aspects of their teaching.

When working towards the development of physical literacy the interaction of the practitioner with the participants is critical. At root, practitioners must be sensitive, responsive and flexible. They need to be alert to participants' responses and able to adapt and redirect tasks as appropriate. As far as possible, participants should be involved in their own learning, as the ultimate goal of work to enhance physical literacy sees participants as having the motivation to continue with physical activity without the need for specific guidance from a practitioner. This chapter has focused on the '*how*' of interactions to foster physical literacy. Chapter 15 looks at the '*what*'; that is, activity contexts that will provide opportunities for many of the attributes of this capability to be developed.

Recommended reading

Fox, K.R. (1997) *The Physical Self*. Human Kinetics, pp. 192–199.
These pages list recommendations for participant/practitioner interaction to promote self-esteem. They are very pertinent to fostering physical literacy.

Graham, G., Holt/Hale, S. and Parker, M. (2009) *Children Moving: A Reflective Approach to Teaching Physical Education* (8th edn). McGraw-Hill, New York, Chs 7–15.
This book develops a reflective approach to developmental physical education. These chapters consider some of the teaching skills and strategies that should be part of any practitioner's repertoire.

Pollard, A. (2008) *Reflective Teaching: Evidence-informed Professional Practice* (3rd edn). Continuum, London, Chs 6, 10–13.
A useful guide to generic teaching principles based on participant-centred learning. These chapters explore some basic principles, and a range of teaching skills, strategies and approaches that can be transferred to physical activity contexts.

15 Physical literacy, fostering the attributes and curriculum planning

Elizabeth Murdoch and Margaret Whitehead

Introduction

This chapter is concerned to look at ways in which the attributes of physical literacy can be fostered by the appropriate selection of material in the inter-action between practitioner and participant. What is introduced or taught can influence growth in physical competence and ready interaction with a variety of environments. It can also foster motivation, self-confidence, self-expression and effective relationships with others. In addition, the content and its presentation can ensure that all individuals have the opportunity to acquire knowledge and understanding of movement and of issues concerned with the relationship between physical activity and health. The notions of breadth and balance underpin much of the debate.

Chapter 14 considered important issues concerned with teaching approaches that affect the nurturing of physical literacy. However, these insights did not address all of the attributes involved in physical literacy. This chapter continues with the debate and looks at the way 'content' can play a part in promoting this capability. It will be found that while 'how' teaching and guidance is conducted is critical to physical literacy, particularly in respect of developing and maintaining motivation and self-confidence, the 'what' of the practitioner/participant interaction has signifi-cant potential to play a part in promoting the attributes.

The 'content' of movement experiences is important in two ways. First, in encompassing the fundamental components of human movement, 'content' can be seen as the building blocks of physical competence and thus the material from which this critical aspect of physical literacy is developed. Second, 'content' in the form of a range of structured physical activities provides the context through which physical competence can be developed and celebrated. Confident participation in a wide range of these activities affords individuals a choice of options in which to nurture, challenge and express their physical literacy. Furthermore, this range of opportunities provides a wealth of situations in which many of the attributes of physical literacy can be developed. The first two sections of this chapter look in detail at these two perspectives of 'content'.

Content as providing the building blocks of physical competence

As was explained in Chapter 5, while physical competence is central to physical literacy it can never be the sole constituent of this capability. Physical competence must be accompanied both by the motivation and the confidence to take part in physical activity. Nevertheless, as human movement is the basis of physical competence it is essential that the fundamental constituents of this attribute are fully understood and appreciated. The presentation of the components of physical competence as outlined in Chapter 5 is only one way that movement can be analysed. However, this analysis is valuable and provides a structure within which the developing complexity of human movement can be appreciated.

It was suggested that physical competence can be seen to incorporate:

- a young child's movement vocabulary
- movement capacities
- general and refined movement patterns
- specific movement patterns, contextually designed for a particular activity setting.

The first of these constituents – the young child's movement vocabulary – was explored and expanded in Chapter 9. It is the task of this chapter to consider the other three constituents in more detail. It is important to appreciate that this movement analysis represents a broad outline of movement potential, not an itinerary of movement challenges that must be mastered to be physically literate. In total, all of these constituents provide a scaffold for developing physical competence, and individuals will be working to become fluent in respect of those movement capacities and patterns appropriate to their endowment. The most important issue is that individuals should have a wide range of movement experiences and challenges and that each should be making progress on their personal physical literacy journey.

As was explained in Chapter 9, the young child will normally have the potential to develop a substantial movement vocabulary. This will be acquired via maturation and through involvement in unstructured, guided and structured play. This vocabulary will include such actions as rolling, walking, grasping, clapping, kicking and climbing. Through repetition this vocabulary will be retained in movement memory and, through use in a variety of settings, it will be refined, show development in control and precision, and thus exhibit enhanced quality. It is suggested that this early movement vocabulary can be built on through experience and progressive challenge in the deployment of a wide range of movement capacities and patterns. Movement capacities are the constituent abilities of the articulate mover. It is the acquisition of capacities that makes it possible for an individual to move with increasing effectiveness and to improve and develop their physical competence.

Capacities are categorised as (1) simple, (2) combined and (3) complex.

Simple capacities

Examples of these capacities are:

- core stability
- balance
- coordination
- flexibility
- maintenance of stillness
- control
- use of power
- stamina and endurance
- moving at different rates/speeds
- orientating in space and accurate placement of the body
- proprioceptive awareness.

Combined capacities

These arise from amalgamation of simple capacities. Examples are:

- poise which incorporates both balance and core stability;
- fluency which incorporates coordination, balance and proprioceptive awareness;
- precision which incorporates accurate placement of the embodied dimension and core stability;
- agility which incorporates flexibility, balance and coordination;
- dexterity which incorporates coordination, accurate placement and flexibility;
- equilibrium which incorporates balance, core stability, orientation in space and maintenance of stillness.

Complex capacities

These arise from amalgamating both simple and combined capacities. Examples of combined capacities are:

- bilateral coordination
- inter-limb coordination
- hand–eye coordination
- control of acceleration/deceleration

- turning and twisting on a variety of rotational axes
- rhythmic movement.

Complex capacities require greater sophistication in the individual's ability to respond. The progressive acquisition of movement capacities will be evident in an individual's physical literacy journey. In some cases the simple capacities may feature alone, such as balance in developing the ability to stand. In other situations capacities will need to be mastered simultaneously, as in learning to walk, this needing coordination and balance. In further instances a complex capacity such as hand–eye coordination may be developed alongside those more basic capacities from which it is comprised, such as orientation in space and agility.

In many instances progressive mastery of the capacities will be seen as movement patterns are refined and become specific. For example, in order to jump an individual will need to have developed simple capacities such as explosive power, balance, core stability and placement of the body in space. To jump more effectively, combined capacities will also be important such as precision and equilibrium and, finally, the complex capacities of coping with the effects of gravity, and controlling acceleration and deceleration will lead to an increasingly effective performance at a more demanding level. Similarly in order to catch a moving object such as a ball, an individual will need to have developed the simple capacities of coordination, core stability and placement of the body in space. To catch a ball more effectively or a ball that is travelling more swiftly, combined capacities will also be important such as poise, equilibrium and agility. Finally, to reach an even more effective performance, the complex capacities of hand–eye and inter-limb coordination and receiving and controlling a moving object at different speeds and from different directions will be needed.

Individuals will make progress in respect of their physical competence as they gradually acquire the ability to apply movement capacities. To develop the full range of capacities will require the individual to have both a broad and a balanced experience of movement challenges that draw on the capacities, and to practise applying these capacities within a variety of contexts and activities. A well-developed repertoire of capacities will ensure that individuals are capable of drawing selectively on these, in order to make it possible for them to perform effectively in a variety of activity settings.

Movement patterns are configurations of movement which develop from the young child's early movement vocabulary as a result of the selective application of appropriate movement capacities. Movement patterns feature in all human movement.

Movement patterns may be described on a continuum as general, refined and specific.

General movement patterns

These are direct developments from the young child's early movement vocabulary patterns (see Table 9.1) and include, for example, striking, receiving, running, jumping, climbing, balancing, inverting, rotating and gesturing. The acquisition of general movement patterns is the prerequisite to developing refined patterns.

Refined movement patterns as related to general patterns

Table 15.1 shows some examples of a suggested relationship between these two types of movement pattern. In many cases this development will rely on the application of movement capacities to general patterns.

Table 15.1 The relationship between general and refined movement patterns

General movement patterns	Refined movement patterns
Sending	Throwing, bowling, shooting
Striking	Batting, dribbling, driving
Receiving	Trapping, catching
Running	Sprinting, dodging
Jumping	Leaping, hopping
Rotating	Turning, spinning

Specific movement patterns as related to refined movement patterns

When refined movement patterns are drawn on in the context of specific physical activities, they need to be further developed in line with the demands and rules of the situation. Specific patterns will need to be honed through the application of movement capacities. For example,
In cricket:

- bowling becomes overarm bowling;
- batting can become the forward drive;
- trapping becomes a part of wicket keeping.

In football:

- trapping can become 'chest trapping';
- driving can become the 'out-side foot pass';
- shooting can become 'heading'.

In athletics:

- throwing can become launching the javelin;
- turning can become part of throwing the discus;
- jumping can become long jump.

Individuals will continue on their physical literacy journey as they gradually acquire the ability to perform ever more refined and specific movement patterns. Importantly, individuals should have experience of a wide range of patterns including: those focused on management of the embodied dimension; those demanding interaction with both fixed objects such as a climbing frame and moveable objects such as balls; and those that demand reacting to a changing environment. It is through an individual's progress across a breadth of patterns, on the continuum from general to specific, that the growth of physical literacy can be recognised.

As has been stressed above, an individual's physical literacy, in respect of physical competence, will depend on experience of a broad and balanced range of movement capacities and movement patterns. This is particularly important in childhood and adolescence when the roots of physical literacy should be established. The responsibility for this broad and balanced experience will lie with parents, carers and teachers. Parents and carers are in a position to promote participation of young people in a wide variety of contexts, possibly encouraging them to take up opportunities offered in extra-curricular time and/or taking steps to enroll these youngsters on activity schemes out of school. However, it would be true to say that it is teachers who will have the principal responsibility for ensuring a thorough grounding in the movement capacities and movement patterns.[1]

The analysis of movement suggested above is one way of describing the constituents of movement. This is not intended to be the definitive method of analysis and there are a number of other systems that are worthy of consideration.[2] However, what is proposed here is a comprehensive, progressive and developmental system that facilitates the creation and description of individual profiles of movement competence, related to personal endowment. The critical point to make is that, for individuals to develop physical competence, they need to experience and work to master progressively challenging demands. This is true for all, whatever their endowment. All progress, however small and on whatever level, should be celebrated. Any system of movement analysis will provide a framework that supports and guides movement experiences through which physical competence can be developed.

Content as providing a broad experience of a range of structured physical activity settings

As was indicated in Chapter 5, another value of acquiring a wide range of movement capacities and movement patterns is that this will facilitate easier access to a variety of structured physical activity settings.

These contexts are important as they provide opportunities for individuals to develop other attributes of physical literacy such as motivation, confidence, self-expression and effective relationships with others. All aspects of physical competence will be enhanced through experience in different activity settings on account of the need for movement patterns to be progressively refined to meet the particular challenge of the activity. This is a significant reason why a range of settings should be experienced, as only in this way will the numerous movement patterns and related movement capacities be further challenged. There is, in fact, a reciprocal relationship between movement capacities, movement patterns and activity settings, as it is very often the case that progressive refinement of movement capacities and patterns is in the interests of effective involvement in structured physical activity settings.

Breadth and balance are key. Not only should participants experience a range of contexts for physical activity, they should also have sufficient time to become familiar with these different settings. Participants need to appreciate fully the expectations, demands and potential satisfaction that can arise from within each setting. The attribute of physical literacy that refers to effective interaction with a range of environments and the ability to 'read' the features in the world around will also be fostered through the experience of interacting with a variety of environments in a range of activity settings. This variety was exemplified in Chapter 5 in discussing physically challenging situations. The suggestions below build from this earlier explanation. It is highly desirable for participants to be involved in a wide range of structured physical activities, these taking place in very different contexts: indoors, outdoors, alone, with others, and in both predictable and unpredictable situations.

To ensure breadth and balance of experience it is helpful to categorise movement settings. One way of categorising these is to identify different 'Movement Forms'. These are: Adventure, Aesthetic and Expressive, Athletic, Competitive, Fitness and Health and Interactive/Relational.

1   *Adventure Form* is characterised by the focus on meeting risk and managing challenge within the natural and often unpredictable environments.
2   *Aesthetic and Expressive Form* is characterised by the embodied dimension being used as an expressive instrument within a creative, aesthetic or artistic context.

3   *Athletic Form* is characterised by challenges placed on the embodied dimension to reach personal maximum power, distance, speed and accuracy within the context of competition in a controlled environment.
4   *Competitive Form* is characterised by the outwitting of opponents both singly and in teams, managing a variety of implements and objects, and coping with changing and challenging conditions and terrain in order to achieve predetermined goals.
5   *Fitness and Health Form* is characterised by the goal to increase movement ability through: repetition; focus on the 'body' function; gradual quantity change; and gradual quality change.
6   *Interactional/Relational Form* is characterised by the recognition that taking part in physical activity can be a social experience, founded on the empathy between people as they move together.

As can be seen, this categorisation is founded as much on the overall nature of the activity, for example, involving adventure, providing opportunities for social interaction or promoting self-expression, as on the nature of the movement challenges, for example, managing the embodied dimension in the Athletic Form and tailoring movement responses to changing situations in the Competitive Form. There is, therefore, a holistic ring about this categorisation, revealing the multi-layered experience wrought in these different settings. This point will be picked up again later in this chapter. However, this multi-layered experience poses some problems in assigning structured activities to a particular Form. For example, a setting that might be viewed by some as competitive may be experienced by others as an opportunity to enhance fitness, while involvement in another activity could be seen as either an opportunity to use movement expressively or to relax in a social context. The value of a particular Form to an individual often relates to the significance of the mover's intention in taking part. Nevertheless, it is a useful exercise to propose activities that frequently relate closely to a particular Form. Table 15.2 sets out some suggestions.

There are two key points that should be made concerning the need for a broad experience. The first relates to early life, for example, the years of schooling, and the second to adulthood. At an early stage it is essential that young people have a satisfactory experience of a wide range of structured activities. Young people need to be fully aware of the movement demands of activities, the nature of the interaction with others and the characteristics of activities as suggested in the categorisation above. The second point is closely linked to the first, in that, unless individuals have had a rich variety of experiences they will not be able to make informed choices in adulthood. A broad experience will provide real options of activity settings from which to select, as endowment alters over the years.

This notion highlights the need for those with responsibility for creating programmes for young people to look very carefully at the range and selection of activities they plan or offer. Traditionally in the UK, there have been

Table 15.2 Structured physical activity settings in relation to Movement Forms

Movement Form	Structured physical activity
Adventure	Climbing; abseiling; orienteering; skiing; skating; swimming strokes
Aesthetic and Expressive	Dance: modern, contemporary, jazz, ballet, tap; rhythmic gymnastics
Athletic	Gymnastics; track and field: javelin, discus, pentathalon, mile, relays, high jump, long jump, triple jump, hurdling
Competitive	Football; cricket; netball; bowls; volleyball; rugby; archery
Fitness and Health	Aerobics; pilates; circuits; rambling
Interactive/Relational	Dance: country, line, folk, social; synchronised swimming

some moves towards breadth but less concern to address balance. Competitive and athletic forms have tended to dominate the school curriculum and extra-curricular time. Activities from other Forms have sometimes been experienced but in many cases considerably less time has been given to them. This would include Adventure, Aesthetic and Expressive, Fitness and Health and Interactive/Relational. This is very unfortunate on two counts. It means, first, that movement capacities and movement patterns used predominantly in the less favoured activities are inadequately addressed and effective interaction with these environments is not established. Second, for those young people who, for a variety of reasons, do not gain any satisfaction from Competitive and Athletic Forms, it will mean that they will not have had sufficient experience to realise their potential in other activities. Motivation in respect of participation may have been lost and it is doubtful if these young people will continue to be physically active once schooling is over.

In constructing a curriculum or planning movement opportunities those with responsibility need to review the different activity content options and select a range that includes activities from each Movement Form. Participation in each Form provides a distinctive and unique experience that cannot be replicated by involvement in another Form. Participants need to experience activities from each Movement Form so that they are aware of the particular challenges and opportunities each offers. To omit experience from within one Form would deprive the individual of the personal knowledge of the characteristics of that Form. It would also give participants less opportunity to develop certain attributes of physical literacy. For example, a lack of opportunities from within the Aesthetic and Expressive

Form would mean that participants have little chance to develop self-expression, and lack of experience in challenging outdoor situations would mean that individuals have little opportunity to face unpredictable settings wherein they can develop independence and self-confidence. All young people should have a breadth of experience to enable them to find preferred avenues to express their physical literacy and thus enable them to make an informed choice in future years.

In the restrictions common within school curricula, practitioners should use extra-curricular time wisely, introducing more opportunities for students to experience activities from all Movement Forms. Participation in extra-curricular activities should be seen as an exciting opportunity for all to experience new activities. The long-established association of extra-curricular work as being only for the most gifted is unfortunate and deprives many of broadening their experience of a range of activities. In planning curricular and extra curricular programmes practitioners should look in depth at the contribution activities can make to developing physical literacy. An exercise exemplified in Table 15.3 would be useful in devising such programmes.

Finally, it is useful to reiterate how a broad and balanced experience of activities will ensure that all the attributes of physical literacy can be fostered. By involvement in activities from all the Movement Forms, participants will have the opportunity to:

- develop of a range of specific movement patterns and their constituent movement capacities, thereby enhancing *movement competence and confidence and self-esteem*;
- have experience of a range of environments in which to develop *effective interaction*;
- have experience of working alongside others in different ways to nurture *interpersonal understanding and empathy*;
- have experience of using initiative and imagination in interacting with unpredictable environments, thereby encouraging *self-confidence and independence*;
- have experience of using movement as an *expressive* medium;
- have firsthand experience of coming to appreciate *embodied health*.

Motivation and lifelong participation

With motivation at the heart of physical literacy it is useful to rehearse again the ways in which this interest and commitment can be promoted. Motivation will usually arise as a result of recognised personal improvement in respect of movement competence in particular environments. It will be most readily realised in activity contexts in which the participant feels 'at home', and this is likely to be in situations in which the individual is making

Table 15.3 Relationships between structured physical activities, attributes of physical literacy, movement components and contexts and individual needs/interests

Activity	Movement Form	Attributes of physical literacy addressed	Movement capacities/ movement patterns	Context e.g.	Needs/interests that could be fulfilled e.g.
Hockey	Competitive	e.g. physical competence, 'reading' the environment, self-assurance	Capacities, e.g. use of power, moving at different speeds, hand–eye coordination; Patterns, e.g. dribbling, shooting, dodging	Outdoor, unpredictable and challenging environment	Competitive urge, belonging to a group – social interaction, fitness
Dance	Aesthetic and Expressive	e.g. physical competence, self-awareness, ability to express self and interact with empathy	Capacities, e.g. poise, control, fluency; Patterns, e.g. turning, leaping, spinning	Indoor, musical accompaniment, no apparatus or equipment	Self-expression, exploration of movement in an aesthetic context, moving with others, relaxation from work stress, fitness
Pilates	Health and Fitness	e.g. physical competence, understanding of embodied health	Capacities, e.g. flexibility, balance, precision; Patterns, e.g. rolling, curling, stretching	Indoor, no equipment, predictable environment	Health and fitness, relaxation from work stress

progress and achieving success. In addition, motivation to take part will be strengthened if participation fulfils a personal need. It may be the case that the individual is not overly successful in a certain activity context; however, because participation fulfils a need, this context may become the preferred activity area. For example, the decision to take part in an activity may arise from:

- the pure enjoyment of successful participation;
- the excitement of competitive situations;
- an appetite to experience and master new challenges;
- the enjoyment and satisfaction of moving in an aesthetic context;
- the exhilaration of beating personal goals in respect of, for example, strength or speed;
- the determination to match up to and beat others;
- social needs to be with others;
- a personal need to relax away from the stress of a job;
- a strong desire to become fitter or lose weight;
- a love of the countryside.

Any of these are quite legitimate reasons for taking part in physical activity. It is perhaps the case that this very acceptable range of needs and interests are not made clear to young people. There is a generally accepted view that the only legitimate reason to be involved in physical activity is because an individual is highly skilled and can be 'a winner'. Where individuals can see no possibility of excelling in comparison with others there can seem to be no reason for them to participate. This is an unfortunate situation given the range of needs that participation in physical activity can fulfil. Of course personal needs can also be met by involvement in numerous other activities and pursuits, from singing in a choir to playing chess, and from attending operatic performances to stamp collecting. However, being physically literate gives individuals the option of fulfilling personal needs in the context of physical activity.

Knowledge and understanding of movement and of the relationship between physical activity and health

In considering how the material or 'content' of the interaction between participants and practitioners can address the attributes of physical literacy, the final aspect to be covered is the development of knowledge and understanding of movement and of embodied health. An understanding of the nature of movement, of its constituents and how these constituents can be combined, is probably best introduced as the participant is engaged in exploring and developing movement capacities and movement patterns. In a sense this may be seen as part of the teaching approach adopted by the practitioner. The use by the practitioner of a rich, descriptive language will pave the way for an appreciation of the nature of movement and this can usefully be followed by the expectation that the participants themselves use this language in evaluating their own and others' movement. The use of appropriate questioning by the practitioner and the deployment of methods of recording movement that become the focus of subsequent discussion are both ways of encouraging use of movement language. Knowledge and understanding of movement are best fostered in the context of a wide range of structured activity settings and through teaching approaches that incorporate observation, analysis, description and evaluation on the part of the participant.[3]

Methods to acquire knowledge and understanding of the relationship between physical activity and health have long been debated. Two very different approaches have been advocated. In one approach health and fitness issues are delivered in discrete modules or lessons. In the other approach these issues are covered as movement learning is taking place; in other words, coverage of the information permeates all interactions between the practitioner and the participants. It is suggested that a combination of the two approaches can be the most effective. Disadvantages of the discrete approach alone are that the work can become purely theoretical or be seen as of a different order to other types of learning in the movement field. However, the advantage of this approach is that there is no danger that it is overlooked. The advantages of the permeation approach are, first, that movement experiences themselves can reveal some of the principles of the effect of movement on 'body' systems and thereby on health and fitness, thus making understanding immediate to the movers. With respect to developing positive attitudes to health-related exercise Harris (2001: 2) asserts that 'the most appropriate teaching approaches involve learning through active participation in purposeful physical activity'. Second, through this approach the close relationship of health issues and participation is readily endorsed. The danger of this approach is that health issues can be lost in the range of movement challenges being explored. It is, however, important that this knowledge and understanding is fostered in a way that will equip younger people with the appreciation of embodied health and the benefits of exercise, which they can take with them into later life.

Individuals on their physical literacy journey will make progress as they gradually acquire more detailed knowledge and information concerning both the nature of movement and the relationship between physical activity and health. It is the responsibility of all significant others in contact with the young to ensure that this occurs and it is a responsibility of the participants themselves, as they mature, to keep abreast with new research and information in this field.

Conclusion

This chapter has been concerned to make a case for a rich experience both of the movement components of physical competence, such as movement capacities and movement patterns, and of activities from different Movement Forms. Breadth of experience is essential to develop the motivation, confidence and physical competence that are at the heart of physical literacy. The chapter has also shown how involvement in activities from all Movement Forms can make a valuable contribution to fostering the attributes of effective interaction with the environment, self-expression and sensitive interaction with others. In addition, approaches to fostering the knowledge and understanding attribute have be outlined.

Recommended reading

Killingbeck, M., Bowler, M., Golding, D. and Gammon, P. (2007) Physical education and physical literacy. *Physical Education Matters*, 2, 2 pp. 20–24.

Maude, M. and Whitehead, M.E. (2003) *Observing Children Moving*. CDRom 16672 afPE.

Maude, M. and Whitehead, M.E. (2007) *Observing and Analysing Learners' Movement*. CDRom 023 afPE.

These two CDRoms are designed to support movement observation and analysis. See Bibliography for website details relating to CDRoms.

N.B. Some of the tables from this chapter as well as some additional tables are available on the website www.physical-literacy.org.uk

16 Conclusion and the way ahead

Margaret Whitehead

The concept of physical literacy

The concept of physical literacy highlights the central importance of the embodied dimension in human life. Physical literacy describes the human capability springing from capitalising on embodied potential. The findings arising from investigating embodied potential provide the rationale for arguing for the value of becoming physically literate. Physically literate individuals are in a position to benefit in a variety of significant ways from nurturing this aspect of personhood.

A central characteristic of physical literacy is that it encompasses both the familiar 'body-as-object' mode of embodiment and the 'body-as-lived' mode, the latter being, heretofore, overlooked by many. The concept of physical literacy relies on an appreciation of the way in which the embodiment-as-instrument and the embodiment-as-lived work inseparably to realise our human nature. This claim is founded on the insights of existentialists and phenomenologists who assert that humans are, by nature, beings-in-the-world. Individuals create themselves as they interact with their surroundings. Without the capabilities humans possess to perceive and interact with the world there would be no life. All those capabilities through which humans interact with the world are, therefore, both critical and indispensable in making life as we know it a reality. The embodied dimension, central to the capability of physical literacy, is, in the view of these philosophers, absolutely essential for effective interaction with the world. It is of interest to note that this interaction, as a persistent feature of life, is occurring simultaneously on pre-conscious and conscious levels. The embodiment in both modes is implicated in this ongoing process.

The philosophers' commitment to the all-pervading value of the embodied dimension is in clear opposition to those who see the embodiment as inferior to human mental faculties. This latter attitude to the embodied dimension arises from the philosophy of dualism; that is, a presumption that human beings comprise two separable parts: the 'body' and the 'mind', with the 'mind' being seen as far superior to the 'body'. Existentialists and phenomenologists reject dualism and support a monist approach to existence. Monism is a belief that each individual is an indivisible whole with all human dimensions being intricately interdependent. No dimension is superior or inferior to any other as all function collaboratively, affecting, influencing and supporting each other. In respect of discussions of physical literacy, with its roots firmly in monism, the use of the term 'body' is misleading and counter-productive; hence the use of the term 'embodiment' in explaining the concept.

It can be seen from the brief discussion above that the concept of physical literacy is founded on monist principles, on a belief that humans create themselves through interacting with the world and on the view that the two aspects of embodiment – the embodiment-as-instrument and the embodiment-as-lived – are inseparable and equally important in the lives of individuals. Any discussion of the concept needs to be conducted from a base of these tenets.

The importance of the embodied dimension and physical literacy

From a purely philosophical perspective the importance of the embodied dimension, and consequently its expression in physical literacy, lies in the interaction it affords with the environment. This somewhat general and overarching value has been further developed and specified by the work of a wide range of scholars and scientists, such as Burkitt (1999) and Lakoff and Johnson (1999). As has been outlined in Part I, there is growing evidence that embodied interaction with the world is the foundation for the development of cognition, the acquisition of language and the ability to reason. Furthermore, there is evidence that individuals' embodied dimension is an important aspect of their sense of self and self-identity. Other writers, for example, Gallagher (2005) and Best (1974), have suggested that the embodied dimension is integral to the expression of emotion and facilitates fluent self-expression and sensitive interaction with others.

In short, there is ample evidence that, far from being an inferior aspect of the human condition, the embodied dimension is at the core of existence. The embodied capability both at pre-conscious and conscious levels contributes significantly to human development. With reference to the scholars mentioned above it would appear that a life in which the embodied dimension is undervalued, dismissed and neglected would be a poorer life. This is the assertion at the heart of the promotion of physical literacy. The development of physical literacy, as the realisation of embodied potential, has a great deal to offer to everyone throughout the lifecourse.

The value of physical literacy has been roundly supported by all the contributors to Part II. Chapter 7 argued that the physical self is closely related to the global self, and that attitudes to the physical self have a profound effect on self-esteem. The development of physical literacy, with its stress on motivation and confidence in respect of nurturing physical competence, was seen to be a significant asset in promoting self-confidence and mental health. The insights from Chapter 8 revealed the negative effects experienced by individuals who were not physically literate on account of being overweight or obese. The case study included in the chapter is only one of many that could demonstrate the benefits to these young people of becoming physically literate. There is no doubt that their quality of life is enhanced, they grow in self-confidence, have a more positive outlook on life and develop skills that enable them to have rewarding social interaction.

Chapter 9 revealed the importance of movement development in the early years both to promote physical growth and the mastery of essential general movement patterns, and to stimulate brain development. Chapter 10 looked at adults, particularly the older adult population, and made a strong case for the importance of physical literacy. Fostering physical competence was seen to enhance quality of life, with these older people gaining in self-confidence and independence. Their lives were enriched both through participation in what were called purposeful physical pursuits and the development of new friendship groups. Chapter 11 underlined that physical literacy can be achieved by all. Two case studies exemplified the significant benefits which becoming physically literate can have for those with a disability. Finally, Chapter 12 argued that where barriers to becoming physically literate were encountered by those from a range of particular groups, this can have a range of unfortunate effects, such as isolation or curtailing opportunities to participate in physical activity.

The way ahead: strategies to promote physical literacy

Given the unequivocal support from so many quarters for capitalising on embodied potential in the form of fostering physical literacy, it is alarming that there is so much within Western culture that is hampering the development of this capability in every individual throughout the lifecourse. A range of writers, including those who have contributed to Part II of this text, have offered insights into the nature of the problems that are inhibiting the development of the capability. The list below, arising out of these insights, offers proposals that could redress the negative impact of attitudes and practices which permeate much of the Western world.

The development of physical literacy could be more readily fostered by:

- Promoting a better understanding of the nature and significance of the concept of physical literacy, particularly in practitioners working in the field of physical activity.
- Establishing an understanding of the holistic nature of the individual, challenging the dualist view that our embodied dimension is of little import.
- Working to establish monist terminology that moves away from labelling the embodied dimension as a thing or an object.

- Overcoming the tendency for individuals to perceive themselves predominantly in terms of their embodiment-as-object.
- Challenging the assumption that physical activity is only for the physically talented.
- Fostering enthusiasm for getting involved in physical activity, through strategies to increase motivation for, and confidence in, being active.
- Challenging the all too ready dismissal of physical activity by individuals as of no interest or importance to them.
- Increasing the awareness of parents of young children of the importance of movement, and countering the assumption that children will naturally develop a wide movement vocabulary, without particular steps being taken.
- Countering the growing trend of putting young children in 'containers' for safety, thus limiting their opportunity to move freely.
- Increasing the opportunities for physical play in the life of children.
- Increasing the knowledge and understanding teachers of young children have of the importance of movement development.
- Ensuring that all practitioners appreciate that the fostering of motivation is of cardinal importance in developing physical literacy, and thus in promoting participation in physical activity throughout the lifecourse.
- Ensuring that all significant others appreciate the close relationship of individuals' attitude to their physical self to the development of self-esteem.
- Ensuring that all practitioners understand fully that a wide variety of physical activities need to be introduced to young people, to cater for the interests of all.
- Breaking down barriers in respect of participation in all or some activities by particular groups, such as women and those from different ethnic backgrounds.
- Challenging the assumption that physical activity is not appropriate for those with a disability or for the older adult population.
- Countering the misunderstanding that to be physically literate means that a certain level of physical competence has been attained, and instead that physical literacy is particular to the individual, who is on a personal journey in respect of developing this capability.
- Establishing assessment *for* learning in the learning/teaching situation and developing a proven system of charting progress in developing physical literacy.
- Bringing together all those involved in promoting physical competence so that they share the common purpose of promoting physical literacy and speak with one voice. The development of a spirit of cooperation rather than competition between different groups such as coaches, teachers and sports development officers is essential.
- Reversing the trend towards a high-fat diet and the growth of sedentary leisure pursuits, identified in Chapter 8 as an obesogenic environment.

- Initiating longitudinal research to verify the claim that fostering physical literacy promotes participation in physical activity throughout the lifecourse.
- Improving the funding from central and local government for facilities and personnel to promote physical activity and thus physical literacy.

While the strategies above provide a formidable list of challenges, such is the fundamental importance of nurturing physical literacy that the will to change attitudes and practices must be nurtured, with plans drawn up and steps taken to improve the situation.

The way ahead: needs and responsibilities

Ways in which different groups can play a part in countering problems that are inhibiting the establishment of physical literacy as an important goal for all to achieve include the following:

All those involved in promoting physical activity throughout the lifecourse need to understand the concept of physical literacy, appreciate its importance and be able to explain and support the need for this capability to be seriously addressed. Everyone should appreciate that to be physically literate does not mean reaching certain levels of achievement, rather that individuals are making progress on their own physical literacy journey. All significant others, particularly physical activity practitioners, should work together to achieve the goal of physical literacy for all. There should be no competition between these individuals. Speaking with one voice can be a very persuasive way to argue for resources and time from local or central government. Resources as well as training would need to be available to support the achievement of this goal.

Parents and carers of young children need to be made aware of the importance of movement activity and physical play. Alternative ways need to be found for children to be safe but still able to move about freely. Opportunities should be taken to enable young children to be involved in active play out of doors. Assumptions that physical activity is not appropriate for those with a disability need to be countered. Equally, the value and importance of physical activity to all, notwithstanding cultural differences, needs to be stressed. The avenues for getting this message across could include antenatal and postnatal clinics, children's centres, nurseries and playgroups, registered childminders and the medical and paramedical profession. Resources need to be prepared and a team of experts trained to advise on the use of these materials.

Teachers of children aged 4 to 10 years need to be made aware of the importance of physical literacy for every child. Initial teacher training and continuing professional development must address the lack of coverage of movement work and find ways to ensure that all teachers have the knowledge and understanding required to promote physical literacy. This should include knowledge of the building blocks of movement as detailed in Chapters 9 and 15 and of appropriate teaching methods as discussed in Chapter 14. In addition, awareness is needed of ways to include those with a disability and those from different ethnic backgrounds, as suggested in Chapters 11 and 12. This action is the responsibility of training establishments, schools, those funding and mounting CPD courses and professional bodies.

Specialist teachers, coaches and other practitioners working with students from ages 11 to 18 need to adopt physical literacy as the fundamental goal of their work. This should be founded on a thorough understanding of the concept of physical literacy and the rationale behind its advocacy. They should appreciate the critical importance of motivation, confidence and maintaining positive self-esteem in participants, in respect of taking part in physical activity. This has clear implications for learning/teaching approaches, as set out in Chapter 14. Second, they should understand the importance of offering a wide range of physical activities from across all movement forms as detailed in Chapter 15. For those in school, serious consideration needs to be given to activities offered in curriculum time and extra-curricular time. Steps also need to be taken to encourage and facilitate everyone to participate in after-school activities. These should offer opportunities for broadening experience across physical activities, for developing high-level ability and for working in areas in which competence could be improved.[1] Problems of transport from school to home will need to be solved. It would be in the interests of every child to take part in at least two after-school physical activity sessions a week. Personnel, such as coaches, coming into school to carry out this work should, at all times, work with teachers to promote physical literacy. The focus should be on the individual rather than the activity being taught, with every young person being judged in respect of individual progress, rather than against any predetermined levels of achievement. All these practitioners need to be aware of ways to include those with a disability and those from different ethnic backgrounds as suggested in Chapters 11 and 12. These tasks will be the responsibility of training establishments, CPD providers, schools, coaching associations, professional bodies, national governing bodies of sport and government sports organisations.

Adults should be made aware of the value and importance of physical activity to enhance quality of life, to promote fitness and health and to open up opportunities for social contacts. Healthy eating should be promoted. The concept that physical activity is only for the fit and able needs to be countered, as must any tendency for individuals to judge themselves purely on the grounds of their physical attributes. Adults should appreciate that their attitudes can influence those with whom they have contact, such as family members, colleagues and friends. All adults should be supportive and encouraging towards others participating in physical activity, and avoid being dismissive or negative in respect of the abilities or efforts of others. In addition, consistent messages should be sent out by sports bodies, the medical profession and the government concerning the value of regular physical activity.

The older adult population and staff working in care homes should be made aware of the importance of physical activity and physical literacy, and the contribution this makes to independence, social skills and to the enhancement of quality of life. Resources need to be prepared and a team of experts trained to advise on the use of these materials.

Academic institutions and research funding bodies need to be recruited to support research and development of advocacy material, of systems for assessing physical literacy in the form of instruments to chart individual progress, and of longitudinal research to verify the claim that attaining physical literacy promotes participation in physical activity throughout the lifecourse. Advocacy will be assisted if steps are taken to make inroads into the presumed dualistic nature of human beings. While this is enormously challenging, ways must be found to promote a holistic attitude to human beings, and a new appreciation of the embodied dimension.

Central governments must take steps to counter the current trend towards inactivity and less than healthy eating habits. Physical activity must be represented as of value to all, not only for those with outstanding talent. Incentives to promote activity should be devised and participation at all levels celebrated. Governments should work closely with the medical profession, educational establishments and the media to promote this message.

Central and local funding bodies, in allocating monies for facilities, need to appreciate the importance of physical literacy with the beneficial outcome of participation in regular physical activity. This participation, as has been reported widely in the press, can have a positive effect on reducing crime, dependency on alcohol and other drugs, teenage pregnancy and ill-health. These outcomes are of no small significance in the cost of, for example, policing and the health service.

Endnote

Physical literacy has introduced a new way of thinking about the human being. It has highlighted the embodiment as an integral and crucial aspect of our personhood and has challenged us to appreciate that the embodiment plays a part in life at both pre-conscious and conscious levels. In its way the concept has laid the ground for a new discourse concerning the human condition.

The importance of respecting and utilising our embodied potential cannot be stressed too strongly. As embodied beings this dimension of ourselves is, in many ways, responsible for making us the people we are. A disembodied life is an impossibility. A life in which the embodied dimension is dismissed or ignored can be the poorer in respect of self-confidence, self-esteem, social skills and mental and physical health.

The concept of physical literacy is becoming internationally recognised and a range of programmes have been, and are, being devised to foster this human capability. There are signs that the challenge of the concept has encouraged many to rethink and re-evaluate their practices in respect of physical activity.

Physical literacy is relevant to all human beings whenever and wherever individuals live and irrespective of their endowment. There are persuasive arguments to support the value of being physically literate in terms of *the motivation, confidence, physical competence, knowledge and understanding to maintain physical activity throughout the lifecourse*. This is a message that needs to be spread among all cultures and societies. There is much work to do.

Discussion topics

PART I PHILOSOPHICAL BACKGROUND

1 Introduction

- Discuss the need for the use of an additional concept – physical literacy, that identifies the core value of all physical activity.
- Consider alternative terms to physical literacy.
- Evaluate the varied interpretations of the concept of physical literacy worldwide.

2 The concept of physical literacy

- Discuss and compare Capabilities and Intelligences in relation to physical literacy. See the short paper on the website physical-literacy.org.uk for further discussion of this issue.
- Discuss the interrelationships between the attributes in Figures 2.1 and 2.2.

3 The philosophical underpinning of the concept of physical literacy

- Consider whether there are difficulties associated with accepting a monist philosophy.
- Debate the problems of the everyday use of dualist language.
- Identify examples of the role of the embodied dimension in perception.

4 Motivation and the significance of physical literacy for every individual

- Consider ways that movement concepts permeate language.
- Share with others ways in which physical literacy has enhanced your quality of life.

- Debate the assertion that physical literacy is attainable by all.
- Discuss the problems of achieving physical literacy in Western culture.

5 Physical literacy, physical competence and interaction with the environment

- Rewrite the physical competences for two cultures that would *not* be described as belonging to the 'twenty-first-century Western world'.
- Identify and discuss examples of 'reading' the environment.

6 Physical literacy, the sense of self, relationships with others and the place of knowledge and understanding in the concept

- Debate how physical literacy contributes to your sense of self.
- Conduct an exercise to become more sensitive to one's own and others' non-verbal communication.
- Consider the views that propositional knowledge is (1) essential for physical literacy and (2) inadequate on its own to constitute physical literacy.

PART II CONTEXTUAL CONNECTIONS

7 The physical self and physical literacy

- How can we help people to develop self-acceptance?
- Are we too self-conscious about our physical selves?
- Can we learn to see ourselves as a single entity rather than 'body' and mind, and if so how can teachers help?

8 Physical literacy and obesity

- What is the role of physical educators in tackling childhood obesity?
- Poor physical literacy in overweight and obese children. Nature or nurture?

9 Physical literacy and the young child

- Discuss the key features of quality of life for the young child.
- With reference to the section in the chapter on movement development, observe and then discuss with others the movement development of a young child playing in an outdoor context.

- Discuss the benefits of experiences of free play, guided play and structured play in the promotion of physical competence and physical literacy.

10 Physical literacy and the older adult population

- Debate the proposal that education should be seen as a lifelong enterprise.
- What steps can be taken to make the general public aware of how much physical activity is needed to promote health and well-being?
- What should the government do to promote and support physical activity for the older adult population?

11 Physical literacy and individuals with a disability

Reflecting on flexible movement outcomes

- Sugden and Keogh (1990) suggest that movement outcomes are determined by the interrelationship of three interacting variables:

1   The task to be performed.
2   The resources the child brings to the learning situation.
3   The context within which learning takes place.

Review the three strategies identified by Sugden and Keogh (1990) and identify learning, teaching and assessment strategies you can adopt to maximise learning potential.

The Qualifications and Curriculum Authority (2007) Statutory Inclusion Statement

- The Qualifications and Curriculum Authority (2007) identifies three issues that should be addressed when responding to people's individual needs. These are:

1   Setting suitable learning challenges.
2   Responding to the diversity of individuals.
3   Differentiating learning, teaching and assessment to minimise barriers to learning.

Review the three strategies above and consider how you can use these to meet individual needs and minimise barriers to learning and participation in physical activity.

12 Physical literacy and issues of diversity

The Eight P Inclusive Framework

- Reflect upon the Eight P Inclusive Framework discussed in the chapter by Vickerman (2007). Use the table below to consider what strategies you would use to maximise potential in physical literacy for diverse groups in society.

Eight P Model	Strategies for action in meeting individual physical literacy needs
Philosophy	
Purposeful	
Proactive	
Partnership	
Process	
Policy	
Pedagogy	
Practice	

Equality of opportunity in physical literacy

- Reflect upon the issues discussed within this chapter and identify strategies you can adopt to ensure that everyone has the opportunity to maximise their learning potential and become physically literate.

PART III PRACTICAL IMPLICATIONS

13 Promoting physical literacy within and beyond the school curriculum

- What strategies might be used to encourage all practitioners working in the field of physical activity, with people of all ages, to share the common goal of promoting physical literacy?
- Consider the benefits of identifying physical literacy as the intrinsic goal of physical education.

14 Physical literacy and learning and teaching approaches

- Discuss the teaching skills that would be required to implement the suggestions in the chapter under the headings of Content selected/planning, Organisation and Learning/teaching interaction.
- Consider each of the scenarios from the chapter and discuss how far each represents a context in which physical literacy may be fostered.

15 Physical literacy, fostering the attributes and curriculum planning

- Critically discuss the curriculum outline for pupils from the ages of 4 to 11 on the website www.physical-literacy.org.uk.
- Analyse three different activities in the same form as exemplified in Table 15.3.
- During compulsory schooling, equal time should be allocated to activities from each of the Movement Forms. Discuss.
- Debate the best use of extra-curricular time to encourage all pupils to take part.

16 Conclusion and the way ahead

- Consider the most significant problems in establishing physical literacy as a goal for all to achieve.
- Identify actions you could take to promote physical literacy within your own work.

Glossary

The definitions identified below are those used throughout this text.

Attributes the constituent elements of physical literacy that are identified in the full definition of the concept. In growing in physical literacy individuals will discover that they have the potential to develop all the attributes.

BMI Body Mass Index is the measurement that compares a person's weight and height to determine the overall fitness of the individual. BMI calculation does not actually measure percentage of total body fat, but it is a tool used to estimate what is considered a healthy weight based on a person's height.

Boomwhacker brightly coloured plastic tubes which are tuned to specific notes. They can be played by tapping them against any surface or by tapping two or more tubes against each other to make chords.

Capability the expression of a human dimension by an individual. A capability is a desirable human expression of being, the development of which should be available to every individual. This use is broadly in line with the way in which Martha Nussbaum (2000) uses the term. Capabilities she identifies include practical reason, emotion and affiliation.

Dimension an aspect of human being through which individuals can interact with the world and express themselves. Embodiment is one such dimension – hence, embodied dimension. Other dimensions may be seen as cognitive, affective and social aspects of human being.

Dualism the view that human beings comprise two very different and separable 'parts', being the 'body' and the 'mind'.

Embodied capability the human capability arising from our embodied dimension.

Embodied dimension that dimension of human potential which springs from the ability to move or motility.

Embodiment in the context of physical literacy the term embodiment is used, specifically, to describe the potential individuals have to interact with the environment via movement. This covers both the embodiment-as-lived as well as the embodiment as an instrument or object.

Environment   the totality of features, both animate and inanimate, that comprise the world with which individuals come into contact.

Existentialism   the philosophy based on the principle that existence precedes essence. In other words, individuals make themselves as they interact with the world.

Exteroceptors   sensory receptors that receive information external to the 'body'/organism such as the eyes and ears.

Extrinsic motives   motives that are not integrated into the self-system and do not contribute to autonomy.

Holism and holistic   see monism.

Homophobia   an irrational fear or aversion to homosexuality which can result in discrimination, prejudice and isolation.

Intermodal   see synaesthesia.

Interoceptors   sensory receptors that receive information from within a 'body'/organism such as nerve endings that are sensitive to headaches and visceral pain, and nerve endings that are sensitive to joint and muscle movement and the position of the embodied dimension in space.

Intrinsic motives   motives that are integrated into and compatible with the person's identity and therefore have the capacity to be truly self-enhancing and self-confirming at the same time.

Kinesthesis   interoceptive information that is below the level of consciousness. This information is collated in/by the cerebellum and assists in the control of movement. This is usually seen as a major element of proprioception.

Lifecourse   this covers all the stages of life from birth through childhood, adolescence, into adulthood and old age.

Monism   the view that humans are an entity, a whole, and not divisible into separate 'parts', such as the 'body' and the 'mind'. This is also referred to as a holistic view or holism, again indicating that humans are an indivisible 'whole'.

Motility   the potential which individuals possess to take action in relation to the environment via their embodiment.

Movement capacities   the constituent abilities of articulate movement.

Movement form   defined by the nature and structure of a physical activity as experienced by the participant.

Movement patterns:

    general movement patterns comprise the total stock of movements of which the human is capable. The general movement patterns mastered by individuals may be referred to as their movement vocabulary.

    refined movement patterns are realised when individuals revisit general movement patterns with more specific focus on applying movement capacities, in preparation to establish specific movement patterns.

specific movement patterns arise when refined movement patterns are applied within specific activity contexts and movement forms.

Obesity   a condition where excess body fat negatively affects an individual's health or well-being.

Operative intentionality   that aspect of intentionality which evidences the innate drive human beings possess to interact with the world through their embodied being.

PALs   physical activity levels. This is a tool to compare levels of physical activity across populations. It is a ratio of total energy expenditure (TEE) to basal metabolic rate (BMR). Typical values range from 1.2 (chair- or bed-bound) to 2.0 + (highly strenuous).

Phenomenology   the philosophy based on the principle that we as human beings give meaning to the world as we perceive it. Objects in the world have no meaning prior to an individual's perception of that feature. Objects are only what individuals 'make of them'.

Physical activity setting   a specific man-made environment that has been designed solely to extend/challenge/celebrate embodied potential. This would be particular to a culture and include, inter alia, forms of games and sports, dance, swimming and gymnastics.

Physical competence   can be described as the sufficiency in movement vocabulary, movement capacities and developed movement patterns plus the deployment of these in a range of movement forms – as afforded by individuals' endowment.

Physical education   the term used to describe any structured/organised/ purposeful physical activity within the curriculum in compulsory schooling.

Physical literacy   the realisation/expression of the capability that is concerned with the deployment of the embodied dimension. More specifically, as appropriate to each individual, physical literacy can be described as the motivation, confidence, physical competence, knowledge and understanding to maintain physical activity throughout the life-course.

Pre-reflective   the knowledge/understanding/experiences gained which remain on an unconscious level.

Proprioception   term used to cover all those sensory systems that are involved in providing information about position, location, orientation and movement of the embodied dimension. The two principal groups of proprioceptors are those in the vestibular system of the inner ear, and those in the kinesthetic and cutaneous systems.

Running bicycle   a light, often wooden bicycle with no pedals.

Self   a dynamic system which is constantly reacting and adjusting to life experiences.

Self-concept   an all-encompassing term that summarises how an individual self-describes.

Self-director   the hub of the self-system, taking responsibility for the information-processing and lifelong adjustments necessary to meet the needs of the self. The self-director has two major tasks – to develop a sense of self and a core identity that is stable across settings.

Self-esteem   an evaluative statement about the worth of a person, by that person. An overall judgement made by the directing self of how well the self is doing. A measure of success of the self-system.

Synaesthesia   the way in which all interoceptors and exteroceptors function in unison. This interconnection between the different ways individuals gather information about the world around them is also referred to as intermodal functioning of the senses.

Teaching approach   a practitioner's teaching approach is generally seen as arising from the values held by the individual in respect of work with participants and the purpose of this interaction. A teaching approach is understood to include all aspects of teaching such as management style, teaching skills and teaching strategies. A teaching approach should be constantly under review and be subject to modification as appropriate.

Teaching skills   a range of teacher behaviours, techniques or tools that can be used to bring about learning; for example, questioning, grouping or planning. A teaching skill needs to be selected and used to address a particular goal or focus, building from the teaching approach being used.

Teaching strategy/interaction style   a cluster of teaching skills selected for a particular end. This involves the identification of responsibilities for, and expectations of, both participants and practitioners, and should support the overall teaching approach being used.

Unconscious   used to describe experiences of which an individual is not aware and thus cannot articulate.

VO2 max   the maximum capacity of an individual's body to transport and utilise oxygen during incremental exercise, which reflects the physical fitness of the individual. The name is derived from V – volume per time, O_2 – oxygen, max – maximum.

A fuller glossary can be found on the website www.physical-literacy.org.uk.

Notes

1 Introduction

1 Throughout the text the term 'embodiment' is preferred to 'the body', as the latter identifies the 'body' as a thing, while 'embodiment' describes a human dimension.

2 The concept of physical literacy is not new. For example, it was referred to by Morrison in 1969 (cited in Wall and Murray 1994: 5) and was also mentioned in an English Sports Council flier in 1991. However, until recently the concept has not been subject to extended debate.

2 The concept of physical literacy

1 A more detailed discussion of these two systems can be found on the website physical-literacy.org.uk.

3 The philosophical underpinning of the concept of physical literacy

1 Descartes was living at a time when the unquestioned authoritarian social structures, based on religious beliefs, were breaking down. Formerly these structures had provided all the answers about the meaning of life, an individual's place in society, and the rights and wrongs of forms of conduct. Without this structure, individuals were expected to be autonomous, thinking for themselves and making a whole range of decisions. Individuals had to take responsibility for themselves. In the absence of the certainty of religious beliefs, Descartes set about reasoning what humans could be certain about. The outcome of his deliberations was that the only thing he could not doubt was that he was thinking.

2 For example, Claxton (1997: 223) expresses the view that the pre-eminence of mind on which dualism is founded is now 'philosophically bankrupt and scientifically discredited'. Claxton (1984: 28) also explains that 'A person is not a thing but a process. As George Kelly said, "man is a form of motion". He is not a noun but a verb. He exists by happening, and if he stops happening, he ceases to exist in the state we call living.'

3 Bresler (2004: 30) discusses problems in our language in writing, 'Deeply built into our inherited languages are the remains of conceptual structures in which mind is separate from and superordinate to things bodily, and teaching old words new tricks is extraordinarily challenging.' In later sections of her book it is interesting to read that neither the Japanese nor African cultures have these problems with their language.

4 Matthews (2006: 6) writes that we need 'to get back to things themselves, forgetting any scientific theories about things in question'. He goes on to say (26):

'The prestige in which we hold science, supported by a philosophical tradition which exalts mathematical reason and intellect over the senses leads us to think that the real world is the one which science reveals to us. We have to rediscover the world in which we live, yet we are prone to forget.'

5 The term proprioception is preferred over kinaesthesia as the former includes the latter, as well as other information from, for example, the balance mechanisms of the ears.

6 Gill (2000) discusses Polanyi's work at length. For example, he writes: (51) 'the interaction between the focal awareness and conceptual activity giv(es) rise to explicit knowing, . . . and the interaction between bodily activity and subsidiary awareness yields tacit knowing . . .', and again (54), 'for Polanyi, tacit knowledge is logically prior to explicit knowing. . . . The main point that Polanyi wishes to make is that because tacit knowing is the anchor or tether for explicit knowing, it necessarily follows that we always know more than we can tell.'

7 Referring to this 'knowledge' held in our embodiment, Nietzsche (1969: 69) writes: 'beneath your thoughts and feelings . . . stands a mighty commander, an unknown sage – he is called self. He lives in your body, he is your body.'

4 Motivation and the significance of physical literacy for every individual

1 Lakoff and Johnson (1999) have championed this approach and their work is a fascinating exposition of the way in which conceptual development from a very early age springs from our understanding of the world through embodied experience. They argue that this goes beyond features such as space and time and encompasses areas such as causation and metaphor.

2 Reich (1950, discussed in Burkitt 1999) talks about how 'body armouring' plays a critical role in many Western cultures in respect of expressing emotion.

3 It is very regrettable that movement demands are constantly being decreased in Western culture as more and more 'labour-saving' devices are invented. Every new invention deprives us of embodied activity and erodes an aspect of our humanness. There is an alarming drift towards finding ways to dispense with the use of our embodied dimension. This includes ever more ways to 'relieve' the individual of needing to move, such as by using the remote control on our television. In addition, artificial 'body parts' are being used in medicine and in some cases are being seen to function more effectively than 'natural' organs. There is even debate in sport that artificial 'body parts' may outperform 'natural' joints and limbs. And in the future there is the horrifying spectre of robots, cyborgs and what are known as post-humans. The ultimate scenario could be one in which there is the total dispensation of our embodied dimension and the creation of a wholly mechanical apparatus to keep alive a pool of 'living' nervous tissue.

4 With regard to cultural expectations and demands, it is fascinating to read Gibbs (2006: 38), where he refers to the work of Geurts (2002) in respect of the Anlo-Ewe-speaking people of West Africa. Gibbs writes:

> they greatly emphasize the proprioceptive quality of balance. They are openly encouraged to actively balance their own bodies as infants, they balance small bowls and pots on their heads, and they carry books and desks on their heads when walking to and from school. Adults perceive balance as a defining attribute of mature individuals and the human species more generally.

Gibbs goes on to explain that this physical attribute is seen to have far-reaching implications. He continues:

But this attribute is not merely a physical characteristic of individuals, but a direct association between bodily sensation and who you are to become. Thus your character and your moral fortitude is established by the way you move. Thus people are designated as moral or immoral through reference to the cultural categories that implicate and create sensory phenomena.

5 Physical literacy, physical competence and interaction with the environment

1 Picking up on this perspective, Wider (1997: 131) quotes Sartre's view that 'Thus the world from the moment of the upsurge of my For-itself is revealed as the indication of acts to be performed', while Merleau-Ponty describes our intimate attachment to the world as the 'intentional arc'. Polanyi goes further in describing the way we relate to things. He asserts that 'we interiorize these things and make ourselves dwell in them' (quoted in Gill 2000: 39). Gill extrapolates Polanyi's position, explaining that we acquire knowledge through a process he calls 'indwelling', being a situation in which our embodiment and our environment 'come together as a meaningful whole in an "integrative act" ' (Gill 2000: 52).

2 Johnson (1987) expresses the view that it is a mistake to suggest that an organism and its environment are two separate entities. The characteristics of an organism are developed alongside those of its environment and an organism cannot exist other than in its environment. He refers to the work of Levins and Lewontin (Johnson 1987: 207) who assert that our embodiment and our environment 'codetermine each other'.

6 Physical literacy, the sense of self, relationships with others and the place of knowledge and understanding in the concept

1 Gallagher (2005: 83) writes:

The first exclusively *visual* notion of self may be tied to the later mirror stage, or a later form of imitation. However, self recognition in the mirror is only one measure, one aspect of a broader concept of self. The phenomenon of newborn imitation suggests that much earlier there is a primary notion of self, what we might call a proprioceptive self – a sense of self that involves a sense of one's own motor possibilities, body postures, and body powers, rather than one's visual features.

2 Gallagher (2005: 30) endorses this view, proposing that:

The body image itself can . . . at the same time, be both the result of intentional (perceptual, conceptual, and emotional) experiences, and an operative determinant of such experiences. For example, my negative appraisal of a particular part of my body may, consciously or unconsciously, enter into my perceptual or emotional experience of the world.

3 Gallagher (2005: 75) explains that 'In an intermodal system, proprioception and vision are already in communication with each other.'

4 Gallagher (2005: 232) discusses at length the view that the more we come to know ourselves as embodied, the better we are able to read off nuances of the experiences of others. Again, referring to autism, he writes:

The neurology of 'shared representations' for intersubjective perception (Georgieff and Jeannerod 1998) suggests that problems with our own motor or body-schematic system could significantly interfere with our capacities for understanding others. Accordingly, it is possible that developmental problems involving sensory-motor processes may have an effect on the capabilities that make up primary intersubjectivity, and therefore the autistic child's ability to understand the actions and intentions of others.

5 In his writing, Sartre (1957) indicates both that there is absolutely no relationship between the body-for-self or lived body and the body-as-object, and he also puts forward a strong case in respect of the notion that any reflection on our body-as-object will result in our alienation from this dimension of ourselves (see also Whitehead 1987). Both of these views need detailed examination in the context of work in the movement area in school and beyond.

6 This is a fascinating example and one that could be seen to support the notion that while physical literacy is, at root, universal in respect of both time and place, its specific manifestation will depend on the parent culture. An individual living in a culture that had not developed language to identify the 'body' as a separate entity could well achieve physical literacy without articulating any aspect of this capacity. The historical development of our use of the word 'body' is also referred to by Burkitt (1999). He devotes considerable space to the way in which events in medieval times altered attitudes to the 'body'. He discusses the work of Foucault and Elias and explores how the 'body' was seen as 'a universal, lived phenomenon, represented in everyone. The material body of the individual (was) part of the collective, ancestral body of the people.' This changed in medieval times when, he explains, 'the constitutive subject becomes more central and is seen to be distinct from the body as spirit or essence, the body itself comes to be understood as matter and as a mechanism, or as Descartes put it, an automaton' (Burkitt 1999: 57).

8 Physical literacy and obesity

1 Gately *et al.* (1997) also tested the exercise tolerance of 19 obese adults (four males and 15 females aged 40.3 ± 13.5 years). Exercise tolerance was assessed using the treadmill walking test protocol developed for the National Fitness Survey (Allied Dunbar 1990). Exercise tolerance was low with a mean peak vo_2 of 2.05 ± 0.51 l.min^{-1} or 19.62 ± 5.45 ml.kg^{-1}.min^{-1} for the females and 2.15 ± 1.06 l.min^{-1} or 16.28 ± 8.56 ml.kg^{-1}.min^{-1} for males respectively. Comparing the values with the 5th percentile from the ADNFS (24.5 ml.kg^{-1}.min^{-1} for the females and 34.2 ml.kg^{-1}.min^{-1} for the males respectively) the values for these obese people are significantly lower (20 per cent and 54 per cent for the females and males respectively).

9 Physical literacy and the young child

1 This situation of restricting young children in their movement is very alarming, given that development across a wide range of capabilities depends on rich movement experiences at this early age.

11 Physical literacy and individuals with a disability

1 A fuller version of this case study can be found on the website physical-literacy. org.uk.
2 A fuller version of this case study can be found on the website as above.
3 A short paper by David Sugden can be found on the website as above.

12 Physical literacy and issues of diversity

1 A fuller version of this case study can be found on the website physical-literacy. org.uk.

2 A short paper from Ian Wellard can be found on the website as above.

3 A fuller version of this case study can be found on the website as above.

14 Physical literacy and learning and teaching approaches

1 Technology as a pedagogical resource. To discuss pedagogy and physical literacy without mentioning technology would be inappropriate in this day and age. While the sensitive interaction between skilled and experienced practitioner and the participant is at the heart of developing physical literacy, resources that may support the achievement of this goal should always be considered. Technology plays a large part in many societies today, and therefore its use in physical activity settings should be considered seriously, where there is a possibility that it can enhance opportunities to develop physical literacy. In fact the use of ICT/technology in activity sessions can play a valuable part in promoting both learning and motivation. This may be through, for example, using visual media resources within sessions or using digital recording to evaluate work. Further, to work within sessions, the growing network of social communication technologies can be harnessed to develop specific aspects of physical literacy. Different electronic media can be effectively used to share experiences, plan and choreograph work or evaluate and discuss ongoing projects. Technology can never wholly replace the practitioner; however, it should be used, as appropriate, to enhance opportunities, interactions and learning in the interests of developing physical literacy.

2 See grid detailing Mosston and Ashworth's teaching styles on the website physical-literacy.org.uk.

15 Physical literacy, fostering the attributes and curriculum planning

1 In many countries curriculum guidance is given to support teachers in this role. A very important stage of this grounding takes place between the ages of 5 and 10, sometimes referred to as the primary school years. In an attempt to devise a curriculum that would lay the ground for physical literacy and match the needs of these pupils, colleagues in UK have drafted an outline that may be of interest. This draft is to be found on the physical literacy website physical-literacy.org.uk. In essence the curriculum comprises modules to be delivered over seven years, with each module of 12 hours in length. The modules are of nine types to cover the spread of attributes within physical literacy, including many that focus on developing movement patterns and applying movement capacities. Each module carries a question as a title. For example, 'Can I throw a ball?', 'How can I climb, swing, slide, crawl and balance on apparatus outside?', 'How can I get off the ground and land safely?' and 'Can I send and stop a ball in different ways, accurately, as I move?'

2 Examples of other systems of analysis include those by Rudolf Laban and David Gallahue.

3 See CDRom 16672 *Observing Children Moving* and CDRom 023 *Observing and Analysing Learners' Movement,* both produced by the Association for Physical Education in England. Both resources are designed to support movement observation and analysis. See Bibliography for websites.

16 Conclusion and the way ahead

1 There is a range of issues to confront in relation to the use of curriculum time and extra-curricular time. It is the case that within the curriculum there is

seldom, if ever, time to introduce pupils to a wide range of physical activities from all of the movement forms. This gives rise to a serious consideration of how best to use both of these opportunities for activity. One approach could be to agree on a narrow range of experiences, which represent the essential core of each movement form, to be covered in curriculum time, in both early and later educational settings. There would be an expectation that all pupils attend at least two sessions of activity after school. The activities covered after school would, again, be carefully planned to cover a wide range of experiences. The principal rationale for attendance at these sessions would be to give breadth to experience; however, they could also be used either to give pupils additional support in activities in which they were having some difficulty within in a curriculum area (such as swimming), or as opportunities for nurturing talent. A corollary of this would be to rationalise the content of initial teacher training (ITT) and continuing professional development (CPD), to focus, for the most part, on the core curriculum activities. This would be the case in respect of ITT and CPD for both primary and secondary teachers. Only qualified teachers would teach in curriculum time. Extra-curricular activities would be staffed by both teachers and other suitably qualified practitioners.

Bibliography

**Papers available on the website www.physical-literacy.org.uk.

Abate, M., Di Iorio, A., Di Renzo, D., Paganelli, R., Saggini, R. and Abate, G. (2007) Frailty in the elderly: the physical dimension. *Europa Medicophysica*, 43: 407–415.

afPE (2008) Manifesto. Quoted in *Physical Education Matters*, 4, 4: 8.

AHA/ACSM (2007) Exercise and acute cardiovascular events: placing the risks into perspective. *Circulation,* 115: 2358–2368.

Aitchison, C. (2003) From leisure and disability to disability leisure: developing data, definitions and discourses. *Disability and Society*, 7: 955–969.

Allied Dunbar (1990) *Activity and Health Research, National Fitness Survey*.

Almond, L. (1997) *Physical Education in Schools* (2nd edn). London: Kogan Page.

Arnold, P.J. (1979) *Meaning in Movement, Sport and Physical Education*. London: Heinemann.

Artlies, A. (1998) The dilemma of difference: enriching the disproportionality discourse with theory and context. *Journal of Special Education*, 32, 1: 32–36.

Bailey, R. (2005) Evaluating the relationship between physical education, physical activity and social inclusion. *Educational Review*, 1: 71–90.

Ballard, K. (1997) Researching disability and inclusive education: participation, construction and interpretation. *International Journal of Inclusive Education*, 3: 243–256.

Bandura, A. (1982) Self-efficacy mechanism in human agency. *American Psychologist,* 37: 122–147.

Barnett, L.M., Morgan, P.J., Van Beurden, E. and Beard, J.R. (2008a) Perceived sports competence mediates the relationship between childhood motor skill proficiency and adolescent physical activity and fitness: a longitudinal assessment. *International Journal of Behavioural Nutrition and Physical Activity*, 5: 40–52.

Barnett, L.M., Van Beurden, E., Morgan, P.J., Brooks, L.O. and Beard, J.R. (2008b) Does childhood motor skill proficiency predict adolescent fitness? *Medicine Science Sport and Exercise,* 12: 2137–2144.

Bar-Or, O. and Baranowski, T. (1994) Physical activity, adiposity and obesity among adolescents. *Pediatric Exercise Science*, 6: 348–360.

Barton, S.B., Walker, L.L., Lambert, G., Gately, P.J. and Hill, A.J. (2004) Cognitive change in obese adolescents losing weight. *Obesity Research*, 12: 313–319.

Baumeister, R.F. (1987) How the self became a problem: a psychological review of historical research. *Journal of Personality and Social Psychology*, 52: 163–176.

Bee, H. and Boyd, D. (2006) *The Developing Child* (International edn). London: Pearson.

Benn, T., Dagkas, S. and Jawad, H. (forthcoming, 2010) Embodied faith: Islam, religious freedom and educational practices in physical education. *Sport, Education and Society*.

Best, D. (1974) *Expression in Movement and the Arts*. London: Lepus.

Best, D. (1978) *Philosophy and Human Movement*. London: Unwin.

BHF National Centre (2007) YOUGOV survey, September. Unpublished report.

BHF National Centre (2008a) *Active for Later Life Resource*. Online. Available http: <http://www.bhfactive.org.uk/older-adults/publications.html> (accessed 29 August 2009).

BHF National Centre (2008b) Media campaign for 30 a Day. Unpublished document.

BHF National Centre (2008c) *Moving More Often programme*. Online. Available http: <http://www.bhfactive.org.uk/older-adults/currentprojects.html#MMO> (accessed 29 August 2009).

BHF National Centre (2009) *Consultation Document*. Online. Available http: <http://www.bhfactive.org.uk/older-adults/currentprojects.html#MMO?> (accessed 29 August 2009).

Blair, S.N. and Brodney, S. (1999) Effects of physical inactivity and obesity on morbidity and mortality: current evidence and research issues. *Medicine Science Sport and Exercise*, 31: S646–S662.

Booth, T., Ainscow, M. and Dyson, A. (1998) England: inclusion and exclusion, in a competitive system. In T. Booth and M. Ainscow (eds) *From Them to Us: An International Study of Inclusion in England*. London: Routledge.

Booth, T., Ainscow, M., Black-Hawkins, K., Vaughan, M. and Shaw, L. (2000) *Index for Inclusion: Developing Learning and Participation in Schools*. Bristol: Centre for Studies on Inclusive Education.

Böstman, O.M. (1995) Body weight related to loss of reduction of fractures of the distal tibia and ankle. *The Journal of Bone Joint Surgery: British Volume*, 77: 101–103.

Boyce, T. (2007) The media and obesity. *Obesity Reviews*, 8: 201–205.

Bresler, L. (2004) *Knowing Bodies, Moving Minds*. Dordrecht: Kluwer Academic.

Brownell, S. (1995) *Training the Body for China: Sports in the Moral Order of the People's Republic*. Chicago and London: University of Chicago Press.

Burchardt, T. (2004) Capabilities and disability: the capabilities framework and the social model of disability. *Disability and Society*, 7: 735–751.

Burkitt, I. (1999) *Bodies of Thought: Embodiment, Identity and Modernity*. London: Sage.

Cameron, L. and Murphy, J. (2007) Obtaining consent to participate in research: issues involved in including people with a range of learning and communication disabilities. *British Journal of Learning Disabilities*, 2: 113–120.

Centre for Studies in Inclusive Education (CSIE) (2008) *Legislation and Guidance for Inclusive Education*. Online. Available http: <http://www.csie.org.uk/inclusion/legislation.shtml> (accessed 22 August 2009).

Cheatum, A. and Hammond, A. (2000) *Physical Activities for Improving Children's Learning and Behaviour: A Guide to Sensory Motor Development*. Champaign, Ill: Human Kinetics.

Clark, A. (1997) *Being There: Putting Brain, Body and World Together Again*. London: MIT Press.

Claxton, G. (1984) *Live and Learn*. London: Harper & Row.

Claxton, G. (1997) *Hare Brain Tortoise Mind*. New York: Harper Collins.

Coates, J. and Vickerman, P. (2008) Let the children have their say: children with special educational needs experiences of physical education – A Review. *Support for Learning*, 4: 168–175.

Cohen, C.J., Mcmillan, C.S. and Samuelson, D.R. (1991) Long-term effects of a lifestyle modification exercise program on the fitness of sedentary, obese children. *Journal of Sports Medicine Physical Fitness*, 31: 183–188.

Cole, R. (2008) *Educating Everybody's Children: Diverse Strategies for Diverse Learners, Association for Supervision and Curriculum Development*. Google Books, Online. Available http: <http://www.books.google.co.uk/books?id=ixm W-porsOAC> (accessed 22 August 2009).

Connell, R. (2008) *Masculinity Construction and Physical Activity in Boys Education: A Framework for Thinking about the Issue, Physical activity, Education and Society*. Online. Available http: <http://www.informaworld.com/ smpp/title~content=t713445505~db=all~tab=issueslist~branches=13 – v1313> (accessed 22 August 2009).

Council of Europe (1950) *European Convention on Human Rights*. Online. Available http: <http://www.hri.org/docs/ECHR50.html> (accessed 22 August 2009).

Council of Europe (2003) *Lesbians and Gays in Physical Activity*: Committee on Equal Opportunities for Women and Men, 21 November.

Crawford, A., Hollingsworth, H., Morgan, K. and Gray, D. (2008) People with mobility impairments: physical activity and quality of participation. *Disability and Health*, 1: 7–13.

Dagkas, S., Benn, T. and Jawad, H. (in press) Multiple voices: improving participation of Muslim girls in physical education and school sport. *Sport, Education and Society*.

DCSF (2007) *The Early Years Foundation Stage*. London. Online. Available http: <http://www.teachernet.gov.uk/publications> (accessed 1 August 2009).

Deci, E.L. and Ryan, R.M. (1985) The general causality orientations scale: self-determination in personality. *Journal of Research in Personality*, 19: 109–134.

Deci, E.L. and Ryan, R.M. (1995) Human autonomy: the basis for true self-esteem. In M. Kernis (ed.) *Agency, Efficacy, and Self-esteem*. New York: Plenum.

Deci, E.L. and Ryan, R.M. (2002) *Handbook of Self-determination Research*. Rochester, NY: University of Rochester Press.

Deforche, B.I., De Bourdeaudhuij, I.M. and Tange, A.P. (2006) Attitude toward physical activity in normal weight, overweight and obese adolescents. *Journal of Adolescent Health,* 38: 560–568.

Deforche, B.I., Hills, A.P., Worrington, C.J., Davies, P.S., Murphy, A.J. Bouckaert, J.J. and De Bourdeaudhuij, I.M. (2008) Balance and postural skills in normal-weight and overweight prepubertal boys. *International Journal of Pediatric Obesity*, 29: 1–8.

Department for Education and Skills (DfES) (2003) *Every Child Matters*. Green Paper, London: HMSO.

Department for Education and Skills (DfES) (2004) *Pedagogy and Practice: Teaching and Learning in Secondary Schools Unit 16*. London: HMSO.

Department For Trade and Industry (DTI) (2007) *The Foresight Report: Tackling Obesities.* London: HMSO.

Department of Health (DoH) (2004a) *At Least Five a Week: Evidence on the Impact of Physical Activity and its Relationship to Health.* Chief Medical Officer's report. London: HMSO.

Department of Health (DoH) (2004b) *Choosing Health: Making Healthy Choices Easier.* London: HMSO.

Department of Health (DoH) (2007) *Health Survey of England.* London: HMSO.

Department of Health (DoH) (2008) *Healthy Weight Healthy Lives: Consumer Insight Summary.* London: HMSO.

Department of Health (DoH) (2009a) *Be Active, Be Healthy: A Plan for Getting the Nation Moving.* London: HMSO.

Department of Health (DoH) (2009b) *National Child Measurement Programme: Detailed Analysis of the 2007/08 National Dataset.* London: HMSO.

Dietz, W.H. (1998) Health consequences of obesity in youth: childhood predictors of adult disease. *Pediatrics,* 101: 518–525.

Dietz, W. and Gortmaker, S. (1985) Do we fatten our children at the TV set? Obesity and television viewing in children and adolescents. *Pediatrics,* 75: 807–812.

Doherty, J. and Brennan, P. (2008) *Physical Education and Development 3–11: A Guide for Teachers.* Abingdon: Routledge.

Duda, J.L., Fox, K.R., Biddle, S.J.H. and Armstrong, N. (1992) Children's achievement goals and beliefs about success in sport. *British Journal of Educational Psychology,* 62: 313–323.

Dunlop, F. (1984) *The Education of Emotion and Feeling.* London: George Allen & Unwin.

Dyson, A. and Millward, A. (2000) *Issues of Innovation and Inclusion.* London: Paul Chapman.

Eccles, J.C. (1993) Evolution of complexity of the brain with the emergence of consciousness. In K.H. Pribam (ed.) *Rethinking Neural Networks: Quantum Fields and Biological Data.* Hillsdale, NJ: Lawrence Erlbaum.

Epstein, L.H. and Goldfield, G.S. (1999) Physical activity in the treatment of childhood overweight and obesity: current evidence and research issues. *Medicine Science Sport and Exercise,* 31: S553–S559.

Epstein, L.H. and Myers, M.D. (1998) Treatment of pediatric obesity. *Pediatrics,* 101: 554–571.

Epstein, L.H., Coleman, K.J. and Myers, M.D. (1996) Exercise in treating obesity in children and adolescents. *Medicine Science Sport and Exercise,* 28: 428–435.

Epstein, L.H., Valoski, A., Wing, R.R. and McCurley, J. (1994) Ten-year outcomes of behavioural family-based treatment for childhood obesity. *Health Psychology,* 13: 373–383.

Epstein, S. (1991) Cognitive-experiential self-theory: implications for developmental psychology. In M.R. Gunnar and L.A. Sroufe (eds) *Self-processes and Development: The Minnesota Symposium on Child Development – 23.* Hillsdale, NJ: Lawrence Erlbaum.

European Union (1992) *European Physical Activity for All Charter.* Online. Available http: <http://www.coe.int/t/dg4/physicalactivity/Physical activityinEurope/charter_en.asp> (accessed 22 August 2009).

Farrell, P. (2001) Special education in the last twenty years: have things really got better? *British Journal of Special Education*, 1: 3–9.

Fitzgerald, H. (2005) Still feeling like a spare piece of luggage? Embodied experiences of (dis)ability in physical education and school physical activity. *Physical Education and Physical activity Pedagogy*, 1: 41–59.

Flegal, K.M., Graubard, B.I., Williamson, D.F. and Gail, M.H. (2007) Cause-specific excess deaths associated with underweight, overweight, and obesity. *Journal of the American Medical Association*, 298: 2028–2037.

Fox, K.R. (1988) Children's participation motives. *British Journal of Physical Education*, 19: 79–82.

Fox, K.R. (1990) *The Physical Self-perception Profile Manual*. DeKalb, Ill: Office for Health Promotion, Northern Illinois University.

Fox, K.R. (1997) The physical self and processes in self-esteem development. In K.R. Fox (ed.) *The Physical Self: From Motivation to Well-being* (pp. 111–139). Champaign, Ill: Human Kinetics.

Fox, K.R. (2009) How to help your children become more active. In M. Ganzalez-Gross (ed.) *Active Healthy Living: A Guide for Parents* (pp. 52–67). Brussels: Coca Cola Europe.

Fox, K.R. and Corbin, C.B. (1989) The physical self-perception profile: development and preliminary validation. *Journal of Sport and Exercise Psychology*, 11: 408–430.

Fox, K.R. and Wilson, P. (2008) Self-perceptual systems and physical activity. In T. Horn (ed.) *Advances in Sport Psychology* (3rd edn) (pp. 49–64). Champaign, Ill: Human Kinetics.

Fredrickson, N. and Cline, T. (2002) *Special Educational Needs, Inclusion and Diversity*. Birmingham: Open University Press.

French, J. (2008) Using social marketing to reach the hard to reach. Paper presented at BHF National Centre 2008 annual conference, Nottingham. Online. Available http: <http://www.nsms.org.uk/images/CoreFiles/BHSNC_JFrench_2008_compressed.pdf> (accessed 26 August 2009).

Friedlander, S.L., Larking, E.K., Rosen, C.L., Palermo, T.M. and Redline S. (2003) Decreased quality of life associated with obesity in school aged children. *Archives of Pediatrics Adolescent Medicine*, 157: 1206–1211.

Friedman, K.E., Reichmann, S.K., Costanzo, P.R., Zelli, A., Ashmore, J.A. and Musante, G.J. (2004) Weight stigmatization and ideological beliefs: relation to psychological functioning in obese adults. *Obesity Research*, 13: 907–916.

Gallagher, S. (2005) *How the Body Shapes the Mind*. Oxford: Clarendon Press.

Gardner, H. (1993) *Frames of Mind: The Theory of Multiple Intelligences*. London: Fontana Press.

Gately P.J. and Cooke C.B. (2000) A three year follow up of an eight week diet & exercise programme on children attending a weight loss camp. North American Association for the Study of Obesity Annual Conference, Long Beach, USA.

Gately, P.J. and Cooke, C.B. (2003a) The use of a residential summer camp program as an intervention for the treatment of obese and overweight children. A description of the methods used. *Obesity in Practice*, 5: 2–5.

Gately, P.J. and Cooke, C.B. (2003b) Exercise tolerance of overweight and obese children. *Obesity Research*, 11: A99.

Gately, P.J., Cooke, C.B., Barth, J.H. and Butterly, R.J. (1997) Exercise tolerance in a sample of morbidly obese subjects. Proceedings of the European Congress on Obesity, Trinity College, Dublin, Ireland.

Gately, P.J., Cooke, C.B., Mackreth, P. and Carroll, S. (2000a) The effects of a children's summer camp program on weight loss, with a 10-month follow up. *International Journal of Obesity,* 11: 1445–1452.

Gately, P.J., Cooke, C.B., Knight, C. and Carroll, S. (2000b) The acute effects of an 8-week diet, exercise, and educational camp program on obese children. *Pediatric Exercise Science,* 12: 413–423.

Gately, P.J., Cooke, C.B., Barth, J.H., Bewick, B.M., Radley, D. and Hill, A.J. (2005) Children's residential weight-loss programs can work: a prospective cohort study of short-term outcomes for overweight and obese children. *Pediatrics,* 116: 73–77.

Georgieff, N. and Jeannerod, M. (1998) Beyond consciousness of external events: A 'Who' system for consciousness of action and self-consciousness. *Consciousness and Cognition,* 7: 465–477.

Geurts, K. (2002) *Culture and the Senses: Bodily Ways of Knowing in an African Community.* Berkeley, CA: University of California Press.

Gibbons, S. and Humbert, L. (2008) What are middle school girls looking for in physical education? *Canadian Journal of Education,* 1: 167–186.

Gibbs, R.G. Jr. (2006) *Embodiment and Cognitive Science.* Cambridge: Cambridge University Press.

Gill, J.H. (2000) *The Tacit Mode.* New York: State University of New York Press.

Gould, D. (1984) Psychosocial development and children's sport. In J.R. Thomas *Motor Development During Childhood and Adolescence.* Minneapolis, MN: Burgess.

Graham, G., Holt/Hale, S. and Parker, M. (2009) *Children Moving: A Reflective Approach to Teaching Physical Education* (8th edn). New York: McGraw-Hill.

Grogan, S. (2008) *Body Image: Understanding Body Dissatisfaction in Men, Women and Children.* Abingdon: Routledge.

Gutin, B., Riggs, S., Ferguson, M. and Owens, S. (1999) Description and process evaluation of a physical training program for obese children. *Research Quarterly for Exercise and Sport,* 70: 65–69.

Hamilton, M.T., Healy, G.N., Dunstan, D.W., Zderic T.W. and Owen, N. (2008) Too little exercise and too much sitting: inactivity physiology and the need for new recommendations on sedentary behavior. *Current Cardiovascular Risk Reports,* 2: 292–298.

Harris, J. (2001) *Health-related Exercise in the National Curriculum Key Stages 1 to 4.* Champaign, Ill: Human Kinetics.

Harter, S. (1978) Effectance motivation reconsidered: towards a development model. *Human Development,* 21: 34–48.

Harter, S. (1988) *Manual for the Self-perception Profile for Adolescents.* Denver, CO: University of Denver Press.

Harter, S. (1996) Historical roots of contemporary issues involving self-concept. In B.A. Bracken (ed.) *Handbook of Self-concept.* New York: Wiley.

Havighurst, R.J. (1972) *Developmental Tasks and Education.* New York: McKay.

Hayes, M., Chustek, M., Heska, S., Wang, Z., Pietrobelli, A. and Heymsfield, S.B. (2005) Low physical activity levels of modern homo sapiens among free-ranging mammals. *International Journal of Obesity,* 29: 151–156.

Health and Human Services (2008) *Physical Activity Guidelines for Americans:*

Be Active, Healthy and Happy. U.S. Department of Health and Human Services.

Health and Social Care Information Centre (2009) Physical activity among adults. In *Statistics on Obesity, Physical Activity and Diet.* Health Information Centre, England, February.

Hebl, M.R., Ruggs, E.N., Singletary, S.L. and Beal, D.J. (2008) Perceptions of obesity across the lifespan. *Obesity Research,* 16S: 46–52.

Hill, A.J. (2006) The development of children's shape and weight concerns. In T. Jaffa. and B. McDermott (eds) *Eating Disorders in Children and Adolescents* (pp. 32–44). Cambridge: Cambridge University Press.

Hill, A.J. and Murphy, J.A. (2000) The psycho-social consequences of fat-teasing in young adolescent children. *International Journal of Obesity,* 24: 161.

Hoeger, W. and Hoeger, S. (1993) *Fitness and Wellness.* Belmont: Wadsworth.

HSE (2008) *Health Survey for England 2007: Healthy Lifestyles, Knowledge, Attitudes and Behaviour.* NHS: The Information Centre.

International Council of Sports Science and Physical Education (ICSSPE) (2005) *2nd World Summit on Physical Education,* Magglingen, Switzerland, 2–3 December. Online. Available http: <http://www.icsspe.org/index.php?m=13&n=78&o=42> (accessed 22 August 2009).

Jago, R., Brockman, R., Fox, K.R., Cartwright, K., Page, A. and Thompson, J.A. (2009) Friendship groups and physical activity: qualitative findings on how physical activity is initiated and maintained among 10–11 year old children. *International Journal of Behavioral Nutrition and Physical Activity,* 6. doi:10.1186/1479–5858–6–4.

James, W. (1892) *Psychology: The Briefer Course.* New York: Henry Holt.

Jeffrey, A.N., Voss, L.D., Metcalf, B.S., Alba, S. and Wilkin, T.J. (2005) Parents' awareness of overweight in themselves and their children: cross sectional study within a cohort. *British Medical Journal,* 330: 23–24.

Jelalian, E. (1999) Empirically supported treatments in a pediatric psychology: pediatric obesity. *Journal of Pediatric Psychology,* 24; 223–248.

Johnson, M. (1987) *The Body in the Mind.* Chicago, Ill: The University of Chicago Press.

Kasser, S. and Lytle, R. (2005) *Inclusive Physical Activity: A Lifetime of Opportunities.* Champaign, Ill: Human Kinetics.

Khanifar, H., Moghimi, S., Memar, S. and Jandaghi, G. (2008) Ethical considerations of physical education in an Islamic valued education system. *Online Journal of Health Ethics,* 1.

Killingbeck, M., Bowler, M., Golding, D. and Gammon, P. (2007) Physical education and physical literacy. *Physical Education Matters,* 2, 2: 20–24.

King, C. (2007) Media portrayals of male and female athletes: a text and picture analysis of British national newspaper coverage of the Olympic Games since 1948. *International Review for the Sociology of Physical Activity,* 2: 187–199.

Kulinna, P. and Cothran, D. (2003) Physical education teachers' self-reported use and perceptions of various teaching styles. *Learning and Instruction,* 13: 597–609.

Lakoff, G. and Johnson, M. (1999) *Philosophy in the Flesh: The Embodied Mind and its Challenge to Western Thought.* New York: Perseus Books Group. Basic Books.

Latner, J.D., Stunkard, A.J. and Wilson, G.T. (2005) Stigmatized students: age, sex and ethnicity effects in the stigmatization of obesity. *Obesity Research*, 12: 1226–1231.

Laventure, R.M.E., Dinan, S.M. and Skelton, D.A, (2008) Someone like me: increasing participation in physical activity among seniors with senior peer health motivators. *Journal of Aging and Physical Activity*, 16 (Suppl): S76–87.

Le Blanc, R. and Jackson, S. (2007) Sexuality as cultural diversity within physical activity organisations. *International Journal of Physical Activity Management and Marketing*, 1–2: 119–133.

Lee, L., Kuma, S. and Leong, L.C. (1994) The impact of five-month basic military training on the body weight and body fat of 197 moderately to severely obese Singaporean males aged 17 to 19 years. *International Journal of Obesity*, 18: 105–109.

Light, R. (2008) Boys, the body, physical activity and schooling editorial. *Physical Activity, Education and Society*, 2: 127–130. Online. Available http: <http://www.informaworld.com/smpp/title~content=t713445505~db=all~tab= issueslist~branches=13 – v1313> (accessed 22 August 2009).

Liu, C.J. and Latham, N.K. (2009) Progressive resistance strength training for improving physical function in older adults. *Cochrane Database of Systematic Reviews*, 3.

Markus, H. and Wurf, E. (1987) The dynamic self-concept: a social psychological perspective. *Annual Review of Psychology*, 38: 299–337.

Marsh, H.W. and Sonstroem, R.J. (1995) Importance ratings and specific components of physical self-concept: Relevance to predicting global components of self-concept and exercise. *Journal of Sport and Exercise Psychology*, 17: 84–104.

Marsh, H.W., Richards, G., Johnson, S., Roche, L., and Tremayne, P. (1994) Physical Self Description Questionnaire: Psychometric properties and a multitrait-multimethod analysis of relations to existing instruments. *Journal of Sport and Exercise Psychology*, 16: 270–305.

Marshall, S., Biddle, S., Gorely, T., Cameron, N. and Murdey, I. (2004) Relationships between media use, body fatness and physical activity in children and youth: a meta-analysis. *International Journal of Obesity*, 28: 1238–1246.

Matthews, E. (2006) *Merleau-Ponty: A Guide for the Perplexed*. London: Continuum.

Maude, P. (2001) *Physical Children Active Teaching*. Buckingham: Open University Press.

Maude, P. (2008) How do I do this better? From movement development into physical education. In D. Whitebread (ed.) *Teaching and Learning in the Early Years* (3rd edn). London: Routledge Falmer.

Maude, P. and Whitehead, M.E. (2003) *Observing Children Moving*. CD16672 available from afPE (enquiries@afpe.org.uk), website observingchildrenmoving.co.uk.

Maude, P. and Whitehead, M.E. (2006) *Observing and Analysing Learners' Movement*. CD023 available from afPE (enquiries@afpe.org.uk), website observinglearnersmoving.co.uk.

McGregor, S., Backhouse, S. and Gately, P. (2005) The role of motivational climate on a residential weight loss programme for children. *Obesity Research*, 13: A204.

Merleau-Ponty, M. (1962) *Phenomenology of Perception,* trans. C. Smith. London: Routledge & Kegan Paul.

Merleau-Ponty, M. (1964) *The Primacy of Perception,* trans. J. Edie. NW University Press.

Miller, C.T., Rothblum, E.D., Barbour, L., Brand, P.A. and Felicio, D. (2006) Social interactions of obese and non obese women. *Journal of Personality,* 58: 365–380.

Modell, A. (2006) *Imagination and the Meaningful Brain.* Cambridge, MA: MIT Press.

Morrison, R. (1969) *A Movement Approach to Educational Gymnastics,* London: J.M. Dent & Son.

Mosston, M. (1972) *Teaching: From Command to Discovery.* California: Wadsworth.

Mosston, M. and Ashworth, S. (2002) *Teaching Physical Education* (5th edn). San Francisco, CA: Benjamin Cummings.

Mouratidis, A., Vansteenkiste, M., Lens, W. and Sideris, G. (2008) The motivating role of positive feedback in physical activity and physical education: evidence for a motivational model. *Journal of Sport and Exercise Psychology,* 30: 240–268.

Nancy, A., Murphy, N., Paul, S. and Carbone, M. (2008) Promoting the participation of children with disabilities in physical activity, recreation, and physical activities. *Paediatrics,* 5: 1057–1061.

National Institute of Health and Clinical Excellence (NICE) (2006) *Obesity: The Prevention, Identification, Assessment and Management of Overweight and Obesity in Adults and Children.* London: Department of Health.

National Institutes of Health (1998) *National Heart, Lung and Blood Institute: The Practical Guide. Identification, Evaluation, and Treatment of Overweight and Obesity in Adults.* London: NIH.

Nicholls, J.G. (1989) *The Competitive Ethos and Democratic Education.* Cambridge, MA: Harvard University Press.

Nietzsche, F. (1969) *Thus Spake Zarathustra,* trans. R.J. Collingdale. London: Penguin Classics.

Norwich, B. (2002) Education, inclusion and individual differences: recognising and resolving dilemmas. *British Journal of Education Studies,* 50, 4: 482–502.

Nussbaum, M.C. (2000) *Women and Human Development: The Capabilities Approach.* Cambridge: Cambridge University Press.

O'Donovan, T. and Kirk, D. (2008) Reconceptualizing student motivation in physical education: an examination of what resources are valued by pre-adolescent girls in contemporary society. *European Physical Education Review,* 1: 71–91.

Okely, A.D., Booth, M.L. and Chey, T. (2004) Relationships between body composition and fundamental movements skills among children and adolescents. *Research Quarterly for Exercise and Sport,* 75: 238–247.

Okely, A.D., Booth, M.L., and Patterson, J.W. (2001) Relationship of physical activity to fundamental movement skills among adolescents. *Medicine Science Sport and Exercise,* 33: 1899–1904.

Owen, N., Bauman, A. and Brown, W. (2009) Too much sitting: a novel and important predictor of chronic disease risk? *British Journal of Sports* Medicine, 43: 81–83.

Parker, D.L. (1991) Juvenile obesity. The importance of exercise and getting children to do it. *Physician and Sports Medicine,* 19: 113–125.

Pecek, M., Cuk, I. and Lesar, I. (2008) Teachers perceptions of the inclusion of marginalised groups. *Educational Studies,* 3: 225–239.

Perry, J. (2001) *Outdoor Play; Teaching Strategies with Young Children.* New York: Teachers College Press.

Pickup, I. and Price, L. (2007) *Teaching Physical Education in the Primary School: A Developmental Approach.* London: Continuum.

Play England (2006) *Planning for Play.* London: National Children's Bureau.

Polanyi, M. (1966) *The Tacit Dimension.* Garden City, NY: Doubleday.

Pollard, A. (2008) *Reflective Teaching: Evidence-informed Professional Practice* (3rd edn). London: Continuum.

Po-Wen Ku, McKenna, J. and Fox, K.R. (2007) Dimensions of subjective well-being and effects of physical activity in Chinese older adults. *Journal of Aging and Physical Activity,* 15: 382–397.

Qualifications and Curriculum Authority (QCA) (2007) *National Curriculum Physical Education.* London: QCA.

Ratey, J.J. and Hagerman, E. (2008) *SPARK: The Revolutionary New Science of Exercise and the Brain.* New York: Little, Brown.

Reich, W. (1950) *Character Analysis,* trans. T.P. Wolfe. London: Vision Press.

Reinboth, M. and Duda, J.L. (2004) The motivational climate, perceived ability and athletes psychological and physical well-being. *The Sports Psychologist,* 18: 237–251.

Reindal, S. (2008) A social relational model of disability: a theoretical framework for special needs education? *European Journal of Special Needs Education,* 2: 135–146.

Reiser, R. and Mason, M. (1990) *Disability Equality in the Classroom: A Human Rights Issue.* London: Inner London Education Authority.

Rennie, M.J. (2009) Anabolic resistance: the effects of aging, sexual dimorphism, and immobilization on human muscle protein turnover, *Applied Physiology, Nutrition and Metabolism,* 3: 377–381.

Rink, J. and Hall, T. (2008) Research on effective teaching in elementary school physical education. *The Elementary School Journal,* 3: 207–218.

Rissanen, A. and Fogelholm, M. (1999) Physical activity in the prevention and treatment of other morbid conditions and impairments associated with obesity: current evidence and research issues. *Medicine Science Sport and Exercise,* 31: S635–S645.

Roberts, G.C. (1992) *Motivation in Sport and Exercise.* Champaign, IL: Human Kinetics.

Robertson, J. (1989) *Effective Classroom Control.* London: Hodder & Stoughton.

Rocchini, A.P., Katch, V., Anderson, J., Hinderliter, J., Becque, D., Martin, M. and Marks, C. (1988) Blood pressure in obese adolescents: effect of weight loss. *Pediatrics,* 82: 16–23.

Ross, R. and Janssen, I. (1999) Is abdominal fat preferentially reduced in response to exercise-induced weight loss? *Medicine Science Sport and Exercise,* 31: S568–S572.

Ryle, G. (1949) *The Concept of Mind.* Harmondsworth: Penguin.

Sallis, J.F. and Owen, N.G. (1997) *Physical Activity and Behavioral Medicine.* Los Angeles, CA: Sage.

Sartre, J-P. (1957) *Being and Nothingness,* trans. H. Barnes. London: Methuen.

Sasaki, J., Shindo, M., Tanaka, H., Ando, M. and Arakawa, K. (1987) A long term aerobic exercise program decreases the obesity index and increases the high density lipoprotein cholesterol concentration in obese children. *International Journal of Obesity,* 11: 339–345.

Schwimmer, J.B., Burwinkle, T.M. and Varni, J.W. (2003) Health related quality of life of severely obese children and adolescents. *The Journal of the American Medical Association*, 289: 1813–1819.

Seaman, J. and DePauw, K. (1989) *The New Adapted Physical Education: A Developmental Approach*. Roanoke: Mayfield Publishers.

Seefeldt, V. (1993) Developmental motor patterns. In R. Nadau, C.W. Holliwell and K.G. Newell, (eds) *Psychology of Motor Behaviour in Sport*. Champaign, Ill: Human Kinetics.

Shavelson, R.J., Hubner, J.J. and Stanton, G.C. (1976) Self-concept: validation of construct interpretations. *Review of Educational Research*, 46: 407–411.

Sheets-Johnstone, M. (1992) *Giving the Body its Due*. New York: SUNY Press.

Sheets-Johnstone, M. (1994) *The Roots of Power*. Chicago, Ill: Open Court.

Sheets-Johnstone, M. (2002) Introduction to the special topic: epistemology and movement. *Journal of Philosophy of Sport*, 29: 104.

Shilling, C. (2003) *The Body and Society* 2nd edn. London: Sage.

Singer, D. (2006) *Play = Learning*. London: Oxford University Press.

Skelton, D.A., Greig, C.A., Davies, J.M. and Young, A. (1994) Strength, power and related functional ability of healthy people aged 65–89 years. *Age and Ageing*, 23: 371–377. Online. Available http: <http://www.laterlifetraining.co.uk/index.html> (accessed 29 August 2009).

Smith, S., Gately, P.J. and Rudolf, M. (2008) Can we recognise obesity clinically? *Archives of Disease in Childhood*, 93: 1065–1066.

Sonne-Holm, S. and Sorensen, T.I.A. (1986) Prospective study of attainment of social class of severely obese subjects in relation to parental social class, intelligence, and education. *British Medical Journal*, 292: 586–589.

Sonstroem, R.J. (1978) Physical estimation and attraction scales: rationale and research. *Medicine and Science in Sports*, 8: 126–132.

Sothern, M.S., Loftin, J.M., Udall, J.N., Suskind, R.M., Ewing, T.L., Tang, S.C. and Blecker, U. (2000) Safety, feasibility and efficacy of a resistance training program in preadolescent obese children. *American Journal of Medicine and Science*, 319: 370–375.

Spaine, L.A. and Bollen, S.R. (1996) 'The bigger they come . . .' the relationship between body mass index and severity of ankle fractures. *Injury*, 27: 687–689.

Sport England (2006a) *Active People Survey 2*. London: Sport England.

Sport England (2006b) *Understanding Participation in Sport: What Determines Sport Participation among Recently Retired People?* London: Sport England Research Report.

Sport England (2007) *Evaluation of the £1 million Challenge*. Manchester: North West Sport England Region.

Sports Council and Health Education Authority (1992) *Allied Dunbar National Fitness Survey 1990*. London: Sport England.

Staffieri, J.R. (1967) A study of social stereotype of body image in children. *Journal of Personality and Social Psychology*, 7: 101–104.

Stathi, A., Fox. K.R. and McKenna, J. (2002) Physical activity and dimensions of subjective well-being in older adults. *Journal of Aging and Physical Activity*, 10: 76–92.

Stucky-Ropp, R.C. and Dilorenzo, T.M. (1993) Determinants of exercise in children. *Preventive Medicine*, 22: 880–889.

Sugden, D. and Henderson. S. (1994) Help with movement. *Special Children*, 75: 57–61.

Sugden, D. and Keogh, J. (1990) *Problems in Movement Skill Development*. Columbia: University of South Carolina.

Sugden, D. and Wright, H. (1998) *Motor Co-ordination Disorders in Children*. London: Sage.

Summerbell, C.D., Ashton, V., Campbell, K.J., Edmunds, L., Kell, S. and Waters, E. (2003) *Interventions for Treating Obesity in Children*. Cochrane Database Systematic Reviews. CD001872.

Treuth, M.S., Hunter, G.R., Figueroa-Colon, R. and Goran, M.I. (1998) Effects of strength training on intra-abdominal adipose tissue in obese prepubertal girls. *Medicine Science Sport and Exercise*, 30: 1738–1743.

Ulijaszek, S. (2007) Obesity: a disorder of convenience. *Obesity Reviews*, 8: 183–187.

United Nations (2002) *Resolution 56/75: Building a Peaceful and Better World through Physical Activity and the Olympic Ideal*.

United Nations (2008) *Education for All: Overcoming Inequality – Why Governance Matters*. Oxford: Oxford University Press.

United Nations Educational, Scientific and Cultural Organisation (UNESCO) (1994) *The Salamanca Statement and Framework for Action on Special Needs Education*. Salamanca: UNESCO.

U.S. Department of Health and Human Services (2008) *Physical Activity Guidelines for Americans*. Online. Available http: <http://www.health.gov/paguidelines> (accessed 29 August 2009).

Vickerman, P. (2007) *Teaching Physical Education to Children with Special Educational Needs*. London: Routledge.

Vickerman, P., Hayes, S. and Wetherley, A. (2003) Special educational needs and National Curriculum physical education. In S. Hayes and G. Stidder (eds) *Equity in Physical Education*. London: Routledge.

Walker, L.L., Gately, P.J., Bewick, B.M. and Hill, A.J. (2003) Children's weight loss camps: psychological benefit or jeopardy? *International Journal of Obesity*, 27: 748–754.

Wall, J.A. and Murray, N.R. (1994) *Children and Movement: Physical Education in the Elementary School*. Dubuque, Iowa: Wm C Brown.

Wankel, L.M. and Kreisel, P.S.J. (1985) Factors underlying enjoyment of youth sports: sport and age group comparisons. *Journal of Sports Psychology*, 7: 51–64.

Weeks, G., Holland, J. and Waites, M. (2003) *Sexualities and Society: A Reader*. Cambridge: Polity Press.

Weiss, G. (1999) *Body Images*. New York: Routledge

Weiss, G. and Haber, H.F. (1999) *Perspectives on Embodiment*. New York and London: Routledge.

Wellard, I. (2006) Able bodies and sport participation: social constructions of physical ability, for gendered and sexually identified bodies. *Education and Society*, 2: 105–119.

Wellard, I. (2009) *Sport, Masculinities and the Body*. New York: Routledge.

White, R.W. (1959) Motivation reconsidered: the concept of competence. *Psychological Review*, 66: 297–333.

Whitehead, M.E. (1987) A study of the views of Sartre and Merleau-Ponty relating to embodiment, and a consideration of the implications of these views to the justification and practice of physical education. Unpublished Ph.D. thesis, University of London.

Whitehead, M.E. (1990) Meaningful existence, embodiment and physical education. *Journal of Philosophy of Education,* 24, 1: 3–13.**

Whitehead, M.E. (2001) The concept of physical literacy. *European Journal of Physical Education,* 2: 127–138.**

Whitehead, M.E. (2005a) Developing physical literacy. Unpublished paper, PE for Today's Children, University of Roehampton July.**

Whitehead, M.E. (2005b) The concept of physical literacy and the development of a sense of self. Unpublished paper, IAPESGW Conference, Edmonton, Canada.**

Whitehead, M.E. (2006) *Developing the Concept of Physical Literacy.* ICSSPE Newsletter, summer.**

Whitehead, M.E. (2007a) Physical literacy and its importance to every individual. Unpublished paper, National Disability Association of Ireland, Dublin, January.**

Whitehead, M.E. (2007b) Squaring the circle – women, physical literacy and patriarchal culture. Unpublished paper, British Philosophy of Sport Conference, Leeds.**

Whitehead, M.E. (2007c) Physical literacy as the goal of physical education with particular reference to the needs of girls and young women. Unpublished paper, Canadian Association for Health, Physical Education, Recreation and Dance, May.**

Whitehead, M.E. (2007d) Physical literacy: philosophical considerations in relation to the development of self, universality and propositional knowledge. *Sport, Ethics and Philosophy,* 1, 3: 281–298.**

Whitehead, M.E. with Murdoch, E. (2006) Physical literacy and physical education: conceptual mapping. *Physical Education Matters,* Summer: 6–9.**

Wider, K.V. (1997) *The Bodily Nature of Consciousness.* London: Cornell University Press.

Women's Sport and Fitness Foundation (2008) Women in Sport Audit: backing a winner: unlocking the potential. In *Women's Sport and Fitness Foundation,* London. Online. Available http: <http://www.wsff.org.uk/documents/sport_audit.pdf> (accessed 22 August 2009).

World Education Forum, Dakar, Senegal (2000) United Nations Scientific Educational, Scientific and Cultural Organisation. Online. Available http: <http://www.unesco.org/education/efa/wef_2000/> (accessed 22 August 2009).

World Health Organisation (WHO) (1997a) *Obesity: Preventing and Managing the Global Epidemic.* Report of a WHO consultation on obesity, Geneva, Switzerland.

World Health Organisation (WHO) (1997b) *The World Health Report – Conquering Suffering, Enriching Humanity.* Online. Available http: <http://www.who.int/whr/1997/en/> (accessed 22 August 2009).

World Health Organisation (WHO) (2009) *Disabilities.* Online. Available http: <http://www.who.int/topics/disabilities/en/> (accessed 22 August 2009).

Wright, H. and Sugden, D. (1999) *Physical Education for All – Developing Physical Education in the Curriculum for Pupils with Special Educational Needs.* London: David Fulton.

Wrotniak, B.H., Epstein, L.H., Dorn, J.M., Jones, K.E. and Kondilis, V.A. (2006) The relationship between motor proficiency and physical activity in children. *Pediatrics,* 118: 1758–1765.

Index

FOUNDATIONS OF SPORTS COACHING

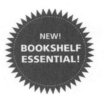

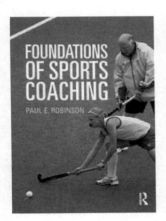

Athletes and sports people at all levels rely on their coaches for advice, guidance and support. *Foundations of Sports Coaching* is a comprehensive introduction to the practical, vocational and scientific principles that underpin the sports coaching process. It provides the student of sports coaching with all the skills, knowledge and scientific background they will need to prepare athletes and sports people technically, tactically, physically and mentally. With practical coaching tips, techniques and tactics highlighted throughout, the book covers all the key components of a foundation course in sports coaching, including:

- the development of sports coaching as a profession
- coaching styles and technique
- planning and management
- basic principles of anatomy, physiology, biomechanics and psychology
- fundamentals of training and fitness
- performance analysis
- reflective practice in coaching.

Including international case studies throughout and examples from top-level sport in every chapter, *Foundations of Sports Coaching* helps to bridge the gap between coaching theory and practice. This book is essential reading for all students of sports coaching and for any practising sports coach looking to develop and extend their coaching expertise.

SELECTED CONTENTS:

Or browse our Sport catalogues
At: **www.routledge.com/catalogs**

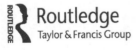

February 2010:
248pp
PB: 978-0-415-46972-2: £24.99
HB: 978-0-415-46971-5: £80.00

For more information, visit:

www.routledge.com/9780415469722

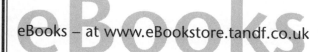